Embracing Diversity in Clinical Practice

A Comprehensive Guide to Gender Identity and Sexual Orientation

Ana Macedo

Ana Macedo

Embracing Diversity in Clinical Practice:

A Comprehensive Guide to Gender Identity and Sexual Orientation

Ana Macedo

1st Edition, May 2024

Copyright © AMM 2024

All rights reserved. No part of this book may be reproduced, distributed, or transmitted in any form or by any means, including photocopying, recording, or other electronic or mechanical methods, without the prior written permission of the author, except in the case of brief quotations embodied in critical reviews and certain other noncommercial uses permitted by copyright law.

Manuel was born a boy. He was a completely healthy little baby with appropriate development.

At 3 years old, Manuel tore the wallpaper that lined part of his room with spaceships and small dragons with a friendly look that blew smoke out of their noses. "I don't like it! I want a castle with princesses, I want fairies with shiny wings and stars!"

There was no problem, Manuel's mother changed the wallpaper. White walls appeared with stickers of pink fairies with shiny wings coloring the environment.

Manuel loved it. He wanted to be a Fairy.

Ana Macedo

Table of Contents

CHAPTER 1 - THE IMPORTANCE OF TERMINOLOGY 7

CHAPTER 2 - A LOOK AT GENDER IDENTITY AND SEXUAL ORIENTATION THROUGH THE HISTORY OF MEDICINE 13

CHAPTER 3 - GENDER IDENTITY 33

CHAPTER 4 - WILL WE EVER STOP BEING HETERONORMATIVE? 63

CHAPTER 5 - DIFFERENCES IN SEXUAL DEVELOPMENT (DSD) 73

CHAPTER 6. HORMONAL AND SURGICAL TREATMENT FOR GENDER AFFIRMATION 83

CHAPTER 7 - FERTILITY PRESERVATION IN TRANSGENDER INDIVIDUALS 111

CHAPTER 8 - TRANSGENDER ATHLETES: COMPETITIVE SPORTS AND DOPING . 115

CHAPTER 9 - HEALTH SPECIFICITIES IN THE LESBIAN, GAY AND BISEXUAL POPULATION 119

CHAPTER 10 - HEALTH SPECIFICITIES IN TRANSGENDER PEOPLE 171

ABOUT THE AUTHOR 203

Ana Macedo

Chapter 1 - The Importance of Terminology

Using appropriate terminology may, at first glance, seem like a minor issue. However, equity begins with our individual and collective ability to use appropriate, scientific, and socially correct terminology that is comprehensive and individually respectful.

Let's start by defining what is meant by sex and gender. When we refer to biological sex, we are considering the body in an anatomical sense and its genetic component. Usually, biological sex is assigned at birth as either female or male, based on visible anatomy.

Gender is composed of individual identity, the expression of that identity, and how both self-perceived identity and its expression relate to the traditional gender roles of each society. Gender identity corresponds to the gender with which a person identifies and through which they express themselves in their daily life.[1]

The acronym LGBT has been widely used in a broad sense, including within itself a diversity of individuals and situations. Constructed from the designations: lesbian, gay, bisexual, transgender; it includes populations whose identity is based on their sexual orientation (LGB) and gender identity (T). This acronym has been modified to include other situations such as intersex people (see new nomenclature for this situation below), queer, or asexual, giving rise to the designation LGBTQI. In a more comprehensive logic, the acronym LGBTQIA+ emerges. Understanding the terminology helps in its correct use and in expressing respect towards people.

We can subdivide the terms related to this theme into the following groups:

1.1. Terms related to sexual orientation

Sexual orientation is defined as the feeling of romantic, emotional, or sexual attraction to a certain type of body or gender identity. The most common forms include: heterosexuality, people who are attracted to others of the opposite sex or gender; homosexuality, people who are attracted to others of the same sex or gender; lesbian people (refers to women or people of feminine gender who identify as having romantic attraction, sexual attraction, or sexual relations with people of the same sex or gender); gay people (refers to people (usually men) who identify as having romantic attraction, sexual attraction, or sexual relations with people of the same sex or gender); bisexuality, people who are attracted to both people of the opposite sex or gender and people of the same sex or gender; pansexuality, sexual, romantic, or emotional attraction to people regardless of their sex or gender identity; and asexuality, total, partial, or conditional lack of sexual attraction to any person, regardless of biological sex or gender.

Typically, the following categories are considered: lesbian people (refers to women or people of feminine gender who identify as having romantic attraction, sexual attraction, or sexual relations with people of the same sex or gender), gay people (refers to people (usually men) who identify as having romantic attraction, sexual attraction, or sexual relations with people of the same sex or gender), bisexual people (refers to people who identify as having romantic attraction, sexual attraction, or sexual relations with both people of female sex/gender and male sex/gender).

The recommendations in terms of terminology are to use the terms homosexual and heterosexual only as adjectives for behaviors and not as nouns that identify an identity.

A person's sexual orientation does not necessarily reflect their sexual history or behaviors. It is relatively common for women who identify as lesbians to have or have had male sexual partners, or for men who identify as heterosexual to maintain or have had sexual relations with men. In this context, healthcare professionals should not assume sexual behaviors or practices based solely on the sexual orientation stated by the patient, although this constitutes a very important element in the clinical history.

1.2. Terms related to gender identity

Gender identity is defined by one's own subjective feeling of wanting a certain gender for oneself. Gender is defined as a set of psychological, behavioral, or cultural characteristics associated with masculinity and femininity. In terms of gender identity, an individual can identify as female or male, on the spectrum of feminine or masculine, or as genderqueer.

People can assume an undefined gender identity, an identity that overlaps masculine and feminine genders, an identity without a gender, or have a fluid gender identity that moves across the gender spectrum, in a continuum between feminine and masculine.

Usually, gender identity is categorized as:

- Cisgender, people who identify with the gender category that corresponds to the sexual characteristics that designated their sex and gender at birth, or as;

- Transgender, people who identify as having a gender category different from the one assigned at birth (at birth, the gender assigned to each child corresponds to visible biological characteristics, namely anatomical sex).

Currently, transgender is a broad category that includes all people whose gender identity or gender expression is discordant with the sex assigned at birth or who do not identify with the female/male binary gender. The designation includes people who live or intend to live by identifying and expressing a gender different from the one assigned to them at birth. It is not relevant whether the person has initiated or intends to initiate the process of transition or gender affirmation surgery.

Gender non-conformity refers to situations in which a person does not identify with the behaviors and social roles assigned to a gender in a given social context. An example of this situation is boys who wish to wear dresses. However, the term gender non-conformity has some negative connotation and pathological sense.

As mentioned earlier regarding sexual orientation, in the case of gender identity, it also does not directly translate to the person's sexual orientation.[2]

1.3. Terms related to sexual development

In terms of sexual development at the biological level, most people are born with typical female or male anatomy and physiology. However, about 1% of people are born with atypical characteristics, either at the genetic level, the level of sexual organs, or the development of gonads.[3]

People with variations in the presentation of sexual organ anatomy have been referred to for many years as hermaphrodites. This term itself conveyed stigma and discrimination. Thus, other terms have emerged, such as intersex people, people with disorders of sex development, or people with differences in sex development.[4] This topic is detailed in its own chapter later on.

Bibliography

[1] Dowshen N., Meadows R., Byrnes M., Hawkins L., Eder J., Noonan K. Policy perspective:

Ensuring comprehensive care and support for gender nonconforming children and adolescents.

Transgender health. 2016 May 1; 1(1): 75-85.

[2] Peter A. Lee, Christopher P. Houk, et al., Consensus Statement on Management of Intersex

Disorders. Pediatrics. 2006; 118: e488-e500. www.pediatrics.org/cgi/content/full/118/2/e488.

[3] M. Blackless, A. Charuvastra, A. Derryck, et al., How sexually dimorphic are we? Review

and synthesis, Am J Hum Biol. 2000; 12(2): 151-166.

[4] Pasterski V., Prentice, Hughes I. A. Consequences of the Chicago consensus on disorders

of sex development (DSD): Current practices in Europe. Arch Dis Child. 2010; 96: 618-23.

Chapter 2 - A Look at Gender Identity and Sexual Orientation Through the History of Medicine

2.1. Early 20th Century

Disparities and discrimination related to the provision of healthcare to people with different sexual orientations or different gender identities stem, from the outset, from the relationship that medicine has established with homosexuality and transgender identities in historical terms.[1]

Until the 19th century, the concept of homosexuality was restricted to describing people who had sexual relations with others of the same sex, and it was practically limited to men. Until this time, the concept of gender identity did not exist. More than being associated with any concept of pathology, the practice of sexual relations between people of the same sex was connoted with sin.

The first movements that questioned treating homosexuality as an immorality and later promoted its decriminalization emerged in the late 19th century in Germany through the physician Magnus Hirschfeld, inserted in the context of the free love movement. It is presumed that Magnus Hirschfeld, in 1923, was the first to establish the difference between homosexual and transgender people. At this time, the scientific community, including mainly doctors and psychologists, tried to develop theories that could explain why some people were sexually attracted to people of the same sex. Richard von Krafft-Ebing,[2] a German psychiatrist, developed the so-called inversion theory, assuming that the sexual desire for people of the same sex came from a sexual inversion in utero.

Continuing this theory, British psychiatrist Havelock Ellis wrote Studies in the Psychology of Sex, a set of six volumes (published between 1900 and 1910), in which the term invert is used to characterize transsexuals and transvestites. In this long work, the author addressed not only male homosexuality but also female homosexuality. The books address the issue both from a gender identity perspective (at the time referred to as effeminate men) and from a sexual orientation perspective. The preface to the third edition of the book, from 1927, begins with the following text[3]:

It has been remarked by Professor Wilhelm Ostwald that the problem of homosexuality is a problem left over to us by the Middle Ages, which for five hundred years dealt with inverts as it dealt with heretics and witches. To regard the matter thus is to emphasize its social and humanitarian interest rather than its biological and psychological significance. It is no doubt this human interest of the question of inversion, rather than its scientific importance, great as the latter is, which is mainly responsible for the remarkable activity with which the study of homosexuality has been carried on during recent years.

At the same time, in the United States, the Society for Human Rights emerged in 1924, the first American organization to defend LGBT rights. This organization was heavily persecuted and lasted a very short time, but it served as inspiration for other associations and movements that were decisive for the current situation regarding LGBT rights.

2.2. The 1930s and 40s - Freud's View on Sexual Orientation

In the described scientific and social context, Freud developed his work. Although Freud followed Ellis's theory, accepting and using the term invert, throughout his journey, he developed his own theories about human sexuality and homosexuality, considering that every human being is born bisexual and becomes heterosexual or homosexual depending on life experiences. Like Ellis, Freud assumed that homosexuality should not be seen as a disease, although at the same time, he considered that it could be "treated."

> *[T]he removal of genital inversion or homosexuality – is in my experience never an easy matter. In general, to undertake to convert a fully developed homosexual into a heterosexual does not offer much more prospect of success than the reverse, except that for good practical reasons the latter is never attempted. (Freud, 1920, p. 151)*[4]

From Freud's work developed in this domain, a famous letter written by him to the mother of a homosexual boy became well-known, in which Freud expresses many of his own feelings regarding the issue of homosexuality.[5]

2.3. The "Science" of the 1950s and 60s

In contrast to Freud's position, most psychoanalysts of the 40s and 50s argued that homosexuality was a disease. Sando Rado (1940) argued that there is no innate bisexuality, as Freud described, and consequently there can be no homosexuality considered normal. Rado wrote that, biologically, there is only one normality, which is heterosexuality.

In a scenario where homosexuality was assumed to be a deviation from the norm, and in which it ceases to be seen as a moral deviation, the attitude of the scientific community was to try to find ways to "cure" it. Psychiatrists and psychologists resorted to (and still resort to) various strategies, including so-called "conversion therapies," electroconvulsive therapy, insulin-induced coma, among others. For their part, surgeons, motivated by Egas Moniz's Nobel Prize (1949), tried the use of lobotomy.

Another practice used was chemical castration, used on men who had sex with men. One of the victims of this practice was Alan Turing, the British mathematician and engineer who invented the first computer (Turing machine) during World War II and to whom the unraveling of the German Enigma code system is owed, making him one of the decisive people in the Allied victory. In 1952, Turing was accused of gross indecency by an English court and sentenced to chemical castration (with diethylstilbestrol), having died in 1954, a victim of cyanide poisoning. In 2009, the British Prime Minister, Gordon Brown,[6] made an official apology on behalf of the British government for "the appalling way he was treated," and in 2013, Queen Elizabeth II granted him an amnesty under the Royal Prerogative of Mercy.[7]

The Alan Turing Law[8] is currently an informal term for a 2017 UK law that retroactively pardons all men who were cautioned or convicted under historical legislation that outlawed homosexual acts.

The assumption of the so-called therapeutic measures was to transform homosexual people into heterosexuals, and after medical evaluation and with family permission, homosexual people could be institutionalized and "treated" even without their consent. Only in the 1970s did the U.S. Supreme Court ban these practices.

In the 1950s and 60s, many scientific works were produced whose objective was to investigate the nature and frequency of same-sex attraction and non-normative gender identities. However, many of these so-called scientific works were contaminated by prejudice, leading to important selection, analysis, and publication biases. These works reinforced these same stigmas and prejudices and created an extremely unfavorable social context regarding the human rights of the LGBT population, especially in the United States.

Some works, however, brought important data about homosexual people. In 1948 and 1953, Kinsey published two books that became known as the Kinsey Reports on the study of human behavior, of men (1948) and women

(1953), demonstrating that same-sex attraction was common in adults, estimated to occur in about 10% of the population (in the United States). Kinsey did not agree with the use of the terms homosexual and heterosexual, having used a seven-point scale that would become known as the Kinsey Scale.

In his report, Kinsey states that about 46% of men have "reacted" sexually to people of both sexes during their lives, and 37% have had at least one homosexual experience.

Regarding women, Kinsey reports that 7% of single women between 20 and 35 years old and 4% of married women in the same age group assumed a score of 3 on the heterosexuality-homosexuality scale. Two to six percent of women aged 20 to 35 reported being exclusively homosexual, in contrast to 10% of men.

Criticism of the Kinsey reports was swift, and he was accused of methodological errors and biases, although his work was based on interviews with 6,000 women and 5,300 men in the United States. The Kinsey Report, Sexual Behavior in the Human Male, became a non-fiction bestseller, selling more than 200,000 copies in less than a month.[9] Francis Wickware wrote in Life magazine in August 1948[10] that to find another scientific book with a record approaching this, it would probably be necessary to go back to Darwin and On the Origin of Species published in 1859.

Around the same time, Ford and Beach published the book Patterns of Sexual Behavior. In this book, they report that in 49 out of 76 distinct cultures that were evaluated, homosexuality is accepted. On the other hand, they showed that homosexuality is present in other animals.

Another study that was an important milestone was developed by Evelyn Hooker and published in 1957, The Adjustment of the Male Overt Homosexual,[11] in which the author disputes that homosexuality should be seen as a disease. Based on her data, Hooker concluded that homosexuality is not directly associated with psychopathology and, as such, is not a clinical entity. This point of view, although contested by many and for many years, would become the dominant view.

Meanwhile, in Europe, advances were perhaps faster. After Lili Elbe, a Danish woman, became the first to undergo gender affirmation surgeries in the 1930s, from which she died (and whose story would, in 2015, give rise to the film The Danish Girl), the first successful gender affirmation surgery (Christine Jorgensen) was performed in Sweden in 1952. Several surgeons and endocrinologists became pioneers in the field of hormone replacement therapy and gender affirmation surgery. However, most doctors were against these practices.

2.4. The 1960s and 70s - Social and political struggles mark medical history

Major changes in the health of the LGBT population emerged in the course of social and political changes in this domain.

In general, there were major changes in the treatment of people designated as transsexual during the 60s and 70s. Hormonal treatments and gender affirmation surgeries were progressively more accessible, both in Europe and in the United States.

In the 1960s and 70s, LGBT movements gained social and political importance. In 1966, the Washington Mattachine Society, which had been founded in 1950 to defend gay rights, made the following statement: "in the absence of valid evidence to the contrary, homosexuality is not a sickness, disturbance, or other pathology in any sense, but is merely a preference, orientation, or propensity, on par with, and not different in kind from, heterosexuality".[12] In 1969, the Gay Liberation Front and the Gay Activists Alliance emerged.[13]

However, this was also a time of cleavage between homosexual men and women. On the one hand, homosexual men were increasingly committed to sexual liberation, and on the other hand lesbian women approached feminist movements, some of them radical. Transsexual people were discriminated against by society in general, but also by gay and lesbian movements.

If in global terms the 1970s brought some calm and advancement of LGBT rights movements, the 1980s brought with it the AIDS crisis. AIDS, which deserved the designation of "the gay plague", was initially a disease unknown both in its pathophysiology and in its mode of treatment. This disease, at the time, often with fatal consequences, triggered widespread fear and raised a movement of discrimination and stigmatization of gay men and those who, although they might not be gay, were socially perceived as such.

One of the struggles of LGBT movements in the 1970s was to get homosexuality to no longer be considered a disease. In the mid-twentieth century, the American Psychiatric Association (APA) exerted great social and scientific influence, led by the psychoanalytic perspective. In the first edition of the Diagnostic and Statistical Manual of Mental Disorders (DSM-I),[14] homosexuality was classified as a mental illness and defined with a sociopathic personality disorder. In DSM-II,[15] published in 1968, homosexuality was reclassified, and considered a sexual deviation.[16]

In 1971, at a time when the APA itself experienced various internal convulsions motivated by the clash between different currents within psychiatry, Frank Kameny and Barbara Gittings, LGBT rights activists, led the Gay is Good movement and explained to various psychiatrists the stigma caused by the diagnosis of homosexuality. At the 1972 APA meeting Kameny and Gittings spoke again before an audience of psychiatrists, this time with the support of John Fryer, giving voice to a "homosexual psychiatrist" who described and emphasized his fear of being professionally discriminated against and stigmatized by coming out.

In 1973, a symposium was held as part of the annual APA meeting, in which the following question was debated: "Should Homosexuality be in the APA Nomenclature?"[17]

The APA scientific committee, called the Nomenclature Committee, debated this topic, discussing what actually defines a mental illness. Robert Spitzer[18] spoke on the topic saying that with the exception of homosexuality and some "sexual deviations", mental illnesses cause anxiety and are associated with generalized social dysfunction with functional changes.

Based on this new definition of mental illness, the Committee decided that homosexuality per se did not constitute a mental illness. As a result, on December 15, 1973, the APA's Board of Trustees voted for the removal of homosexuality from the DSM.

On that date Kameny described that day as one in which "we [homosexual people] were cured en masse by the psychiatrists."[19]

However, this was far from a peaceful decision. Many psychiatrists from the psychoanalytic community spoke out against the decision, so much so that the APA decided to ratify the decision by direct consultation with its members. This situation still deserves discussion today and is immersed in controversy. How can one accept that an eminently scientific decision, which should be based on evidence, can be put to a referendum? However, it is not an isolated case in the scientific world. In 2006, the International Astronomical Union voted on whether or not Pluto should be considered a planet, showing that even in fields where scientific evidence predominates, facts can be interpreted differently and subjectively.[20]

The result of the 1973 events led to the DSM-II having a reference to homosexuality under the designation of Sexual Orientation Disturbance, which classified homosexuality as a disease if an individual with same-sex attraction referred to this situation as causing anxiety or expressed a desire to change it.[21] This new diagnosis had the direct consequence of legitimizing the practice of sexual conversion therapies.

2.5. The 1980s - The path to depathologizing homosexuality

In the DSM-III, in 1980, the designation of Sexual Orientation Disorder was replaced by Egodystonic Homosexuality. More than a decade after the discussion began about whether or not homosexuality should be classified as a disease, and after several changes in the nomenclature and definition of the situation itself, the fact is that it continued to be part of the list of mental illnesses. Critics did not give up and confronted the scientific community with questions such as: should people who feel unhappy about their race or color be considered to have a mental illness? And what about people who feel unhappy about being short, or tall, or thin or fat?[22]

In 1987, in the next revision of the DSM, the DSM-III-R,[23] the designation egodystonic homosexuality was removed and the APA accepted that homosexuality should be removed from the list of diseases and seen as a normal variant.

The following table, adapted from Drescher, 2015,[24] summarizes how homosexuality was presented throughout the various editions and revisions of the DSM.

The International Classification of Diseases (ICD) of the World Health Organization only included mental illnesses from its 6th edition, ICD-6, in 1948. In that edition, homosexuality was described in chapter V - mental illness, personality dysfunctions and psychoneuroses, included in sexual dysfunctions and sexual disorders and classified as pathological personality and sexual deviation. This classification remained unchanged in the 7th edition of 1955. The 8th edition, in 1965, removed the designation of pathological personality, maintaining the nomenclature of sexual deviation. Until 1975, in ICD-9, homosexuality continued to be classified in the set of pathologies designated as paraphilias.

It was only in 1990 that the World Health Organization removed homosexuality from the International Classification of Diseases (ICD-10), stating that sexual orientation should not be considered a disease. However, the ICD-10 makes reference to situations such as sexual maturation dysfunction, egodystonic sexual orientation and sexual relationship dysfunction.[25]

Despite all the advances in considering that sexual orientation can be diverse and normal, this did not imply that the intention to "treat" homosexual people was completely abandoned, continuing to use sexual conversion practices. This fact led several medical-scientific societies to pronounce against these therapies, describing them as potentially dangerous. Among others, the American Psychiatric Association,[26] the American Psychological Association,[27] The American Academy of Child and Adolescent Psychiatry[28] and the Society for Adolescent Health and Medicine[29] took this position.

2.6. Evolution of the classification of diagnoses related to gender identity

The classification of diagnoses related to gender identity underwent marked changes over the years. The ICD-6 classification, 1948, and ICD-7, 1955, made no mention of transgender people. Likewise, there were also no references in the 1st and 2nd editions of the DSM (1952 and 1968). At this time, issues of gender identity and sexual orientation were seen as one and the same thing. In the ICD-8 classification, 1965, the separation of what were considered personality disorders from the then-designated sexual deviations occurred, and for the first time the diagnosis "transvestism" appeared. This designation probably arises as a result of the description of Jorgensen's surgery, where Hamburger, 1953, made use of this term.

In 1975, ICD-9, the term "transvestism" was replaced by two new diagnoses: transvestism, defined as a "sexual deviation in which pleasure is derived from wearing clothes of the opposite sex", and "transsexualism".

In the DSM-III, 1980, two diagnoses related to so-called gender dysphoria appeared for the first time: gender identity disorder in children, adolescents, and adults, and transsexualism. In the DSM-III-R, 1987, a third diagnosis emerged called gender identity disorder of adolescence and adulthood, nontranssexual type.

In the ICD-10, 1990, there was a significant reformulation of the classification and diagnoses. A new category appeared, called gender identity disorders, included in the base category of adult personality and behavior disorders. Five diagnoses were included here: transsexualism, dual-role transvestism, gender identity disorder of childhood, other gender identity disorders, and gender identity disorder not otherwise specified.

In the DSM-IV, 1994, and the DSM-IV-TR, 2000, the third diagnosis included in 1987 in the DSM-III-R was abolished, and the two diagnoses present in the DSM-III, gender identity disorder in children, adolescents, and adults, and transsexualism, were combined into a single diagnosis called 'Gender Identity Disorder,' which assumed distinct characteristics for children versus adolescents and adults. In this edition of the DSM, this diagnosis appeared in a new base category called 'Sexual and Gender Identity Disorders.'

The DSM-5, 2013, brought numerous changes compared to previous editions. The name changed to gender dysphoria. Gender dysphoria separates criteria for children (gender dysphoria in children) and for adolescents and adults (gender dysphoria in adolescents and adults). At the same time, it gave rise to a new, specific base category, separating itself from sexual dysfunctions and paraphilias. Gender dysphoria includes a new specification "with a disorder of sex development (DSD)," which is used for people with DSD situations and symptoms of gender dysphoria. In contrast to previous editions, DSD situations no longer excluded the diagnosis of gender identity disorder. In this edition, a new specification called "post-transition" emerged for adolescents and adults who have transitioned to the desired gender. Finally, the specification present in the DSM-IV-TR regarding sexual orientation was eliminated.

Both the DSM and ICD anticipate that their diagnostic classifications regarding gender identity may be modified or disappear in future editions.

The ICD-11 presents the classification of 'Gender Incongruence' and characterizes it as 'a marked and persistent incongruence between an individual's experienced gender and the assigned sex. Gender-variant behavior and preferences alone are not a basis for assigning the diagnoses in this group.'

In July 2020, the APA issued a statement titled Position Statement on Issues Related to Sexual Orientation and Gender Minority Status. In this document, it states:

"There are diverse sexual orientations and gender identities as part of the human condition. Widespread stigma against those with diverse sexual orientations and gender identities is present in society and contributes to higher rates of psychiatric disorders in these populations. An inclusive and supportive environment for individuals who identify with diverse sexual orientations and gender identities is associated with favorable mental health outcomes (1-9).

Efforts to change an individual's sexual orientation or gender expression have been shown to be harmful and potentially fatal (10-27). Furthermore, discrimination against these individuals can negatively affect their mental health, necessitating intervention by mental health professionals (27-38).

APA's Position:

1. The APA reaffirms that sexual orientation and gender minority status, whether expressed in action, fantasy, or identity, do not, in themselves, imply any impairment in judgment, stability, reliability, social or vocational capabilities.

2. The APA supports the use of gender-affirming and diversity-affirming mental health treatments.

3. The APA condemns any practice that aims to change a person's sexual orientation or gender expression in the form of conversion therapy, or any other similar therapy, as being ethically and morally wrong, and further asserts that these practices pose a significant risk of harm by subjecting individuals to forms of treatment that are not scientifically validated.

4. The APA opposes discrimination against those with diverse sexual orientations and gender identities, whether in education, employment, military service, immigration and naturalization status, housing, income, eligibility for government services, pension benefits, property inheritance, spousal survival rights, family status, access to health services, and the legal right to marry, adopt, and co-adopt."

Bibliography

[1] Socarides C. W. Homosexuality and medicine. JAMA. 1970; 212(7): 1199-1202.

[2] von Krafft-Ebing R. Psychopathia sexualis, with especial reference to the antipathic sexual instinct, a medico-forensic study. Translation published by Rehman, F. J. No copyright; 1852. Available from: https://archive.org/details/psychopathiasexu00krafuoft. [Accessed in 30/1/18].

[3] Ellis H. Studies in the psychology of sex, vol II, sexual inversion. No Copyright; 1927. ProjectGutenberg e-book. Available from:

http://onlinebooks.library.upenn.edu/webbin/gutbook/ /lookup?num.13611. [Accessed in 30/1/18].

[4] A History of Homosexuality and Organized Psychoanalysis. Available from: https://www.researchgate.net/publication/23298844_A_History_of_Homosexuality_and_Organized_Psychoanalysis [Accessed in 3/3/18].

[5] http://www.lettersofnote.com/2009/10/homosexuality-is-nothing-to-be-ashamed.html

[6] Gordon Brown: I'm proud to say sorry to a real war hero. https://www.telegraph.co.uk/news//politics/gordon-brown/6170112/Gordon-Brown-Im-proud-to-say-sorry-to-a-real-war-hero.html[Accessed in 30/1/18].

[7] Alan Turing granted Royal pardon by the Queen in https://www.telegraph.co.uk/history//world-war-two/10536246/Alan-Turing-granted-Royal-pardon-by-the-Queen.html [Accessed in 30/1/18].

[8] Press release: Thousands officially pardoned under 'Turing's Law' in https://www.gov.uk//government/news/thousands-officially-pardoned-under-turings-law [Accessed in 3/3/18].

[9] https://www.cbsnews.com/news/50-years-after-the-kinsey-report/ [Accessed in 3/3/18].

[10] https://books.google.pt/books?id=10cEAAAAMBAJ&lpg=PP1&pg=PA87&redir_esc=y#v=onepage&q&f=false [Accessed in 3/3/18].

[11] Hooker E. The adjustment of the male overt homosexual. Journal of Projective Techniques.1957; 21(1): 18-31.

[12] Graham R., Berkowitz B., Blum R., Bockting W., Bradford J., de Vries B., Garofalo R.,Herek G., Howell E., Kasprzyk D., Makadon H. The health of lesbian, gay, bisexual, and transgender people: Building a foundation for better understanding. Washington, DC: Institute of Medicine. 2011 Mar 31.

[13] Bullough V. When Did the Gay Rights Movement Begin? History News Network. 2005.http:// hnn.us/article/11316. [Accessed in 3/3/18].

[14] American Psychiatric Association. Diagnostic and Statistical Manual of Mental Disorders. American Psychiatric Association; Washington, DC, USA: 1952.

[15] American Psychiatric Association. Diagnostic and Statistical Manual of Mental Disorders. 2nd ed. American Psychiatric Press; Washington, DC, USA: 1968.

[16] Drescher J. Out of DSM: depathologizing homosexuality. Behavioral Sciences. 2015 Dec4; 5(4): 565-75.

[17] Stoller R. J., Marmor J., Bieber I., Gold R., Socarides C. W., Green R., Spitzer R. L. A symposium: Should homosexuality be in the APA nomenclature? American Journal of Psychiatry. 1973 Nov; 130(11): 1207-16.

[18] Spitzer R. L. The diagnostic status of homosexuality in DSM-III: A reformulation of the issues. Am J Psychiatry. 1981 Feb; 138(2): 210-5.

[19] Frank Kameny, Pioneering Gay Rights Activist, Has Died in https://www.npr.org/sections//thetwo-way/2011/10/12/141276633/frank-kameny-pioneering-gay-rights-activist-has-died [Accessed in 3/3/18].

[20] Zachar P., Kendler K. S. The removal of Pluto from the class of planets and homosexuality from the class of psychiatric disorders: a comparison. Philos Ethics Humanit Med. 2012 Jan 13; 7(): 4.

[21] Lev A. I. Gender dysphoria: Two steps forward, one step back. Clin. Soc. Work J. 2013; 41: 288-296.

[22] Davies J. How voting and consensus created the diagnostic and statistical manual of mental disorders (DSM-III). Anthropology & medicine. 2017 Jan 2; 24(1): 32-46.

[23] American Psychiatric Association. Diagnostic and Statistical Manual of Mental Disorders. 3rd ed. revised. American Psychiatric Press; Washington, DC, USA: 1987.

[24] Drescher J. Queer diagnoses revisited: The past and future of homosexuality and gender diagnoses in DSM and ICD. International Review of Psychiatry. 2015 Sep 3; 27(5): 386-95.

[25] Cochran S. D., Drescher J., Kismödi E., Giami A., García-Moreno C., Atalla E., Marais A., Vieira E. M., Reed G. M. Proposed declassification of disease categories related to sexual orientation in the International Statistical Classification of Diseases and Related Health Problems (ICD-11). Bull World Health Organ. 2014 Sep 1; 92(9): 672-9.

[26] American Psychiatric Association. Position statement on therapies focused on attempts to change sexual orientation (reparative or conversion therapies). Am J Psychiatry. Oct 2000; 157(10): 1719-1721.

[27] Anton B. S. Proceedings of the American Psychological Association for the legislative year 2009: Minutes of the annual meeting of the Council of Representatives and minutes of the meetings of the Board of Directors. American Psychologist. 2010; 65: 385-475.

[28] Adelson S. L. Practice parameter on gay, lesbian, or bisexual sexual orientation, gender nonconformity, and gender discordance in children and adolescents. J Am Acad Child Adolesc Psychiatry. Sep 2012; 51(9): 957-974.

[29] Adelson S. L. Practice parameter on gay, lesbian, or bisexual sexual orientation, gender nonconformity, and gender discordance in children and adolescents. J Am Acad Child Adolesc Psychiatry. Sep 2012; 51(9): 957-974.

[30] Where Transgender Is No Longer a Diagnosis Assessed in 10/4/2018 in https://www. scientificamerican. com/article/where-transgender-is-no-longer-a-diagnosis/ [Accessed in 3/3/18].

[31] ICD-11 for Mortality and Morbidity Statistics. Available from: https://icd.who.int/browse11/ /l-m/en#/http://id.who.int/icd/entity/411470068 [Accessed in 12/10/22].

[32] https://psychiatry.org/getattachment/2e35c5a6-8a6b-4f4b-ace8-a1703d9ce367/Position--Sexual-Orientation-Gender-Minority-Status.pdf [Accessed in 16/11/22].

Chapter 3 - Gender Identity

3.1. Gender, Sex, and Other Definitions

When addressing the topic of gender identity, it is important to first distinguish between sex and gender.

Sex, categorized as female and male (woman and man), is defined according to the biological, anatomical, genetic, and reproductive characteristics of each individual. Sex is usually determined at birth or even before through prenatal diagnostic means and is based, in most cases, on the observation of external sexual organs. That is, the presence of a vagina indicates a female individual, while the presence of a penis and testicles indicates a male individual. On the other hand, the karyotype indicates female sex if it presents as 46, XX and male sex if it presents as 46, XY.

Although in most people the identification of sex through the anatomy of the external sexual organs is easy, there are situations of differences in sexual development. That is, during embryonic development, variations occur due to chromosomal, hormonal, or anatomical changes, which cause the child to be born (or present throughout life, even if not visible at the time of birth) with atypical sexual development (see Differences in Sexual Development (DSD) below).

Gender refers to social, cultural, psychological, and behavioral characteristics associated with femininity and masculinity. In each society, the models are different but give rise to cultural, social, and individual expressions that define the feminine and the masculine.

Gender identity refers to each person's internal and individual experience in relation to their body, gender expression, behaviors, or other individual and social manifestations. Gender identity is usually accompanied by the desire to live and be accepted as a member of that gender. Gender identity does not necessarily correspond to the biological sex assigned at birth. On the other hand, there is also no direct relationship between any type of gender identity and sexual orientation.

Gender expression, in turn, translates into the way each person expresses characteristics of the gender with which they identify. For example, through clothing, hairstyle, gestures and behaviors, or the activities they practice. In each society and, above all, in each culture, gender expression takes on different contours and is related to the way that same culture defines the feminine and the masculine.

People who identify with a gender that coincides with the sex assigned at birth are defined as cisgender. In contrast, transgender people are those who identify with a gender that does not coincide with the sex assigned at birth.

The etymology of these designations comes directly from the Latin prefixes cis and trans, which mean "on the same side" and "on the other side," respectively. These prefixes are widely used in the field of chemistry, for example at the level of molecular nomenclature, or in genetics.

Although gender and gender identity have always been present in different societies, it was only in the 1950s that the concept of gender identity was explicitly formulated and recognized in the scientific community. Until then, gender was a grammatical attribute given to nouns and pronouns and rarely used as a human attribute, being in this case synonymous with sex, female and male. The first definition of the term "gender role" is attributed to Money, in 1955,[1] and appeared in the Bulletin of the Johns Hopkins Hospital in a text entitled "Hermaphroditism, Gender and Precocity in Hyperadrenocorticism: Psychologic Findings."[2,3] Later, in 1966, the first references to gender identity appeared, associated with the so-called Gender Identity Clinic at Johns Hopkins Hospital.[1]

3.2. Gender Spectrum

The binary gender structure has been questioned and replaced by a gender spectrum that extends between the two binary poles - feminine and masculine, but allows for a whole continuum of positions between the two categories. At the center of the spectrum, an agender identity is assumed, that is, one that does not identify with any gender.

People who identify with both genders are referred to as bigender, and people who oscillate between identifying with the female gender and identifying with the male gender are referred to as gender fluid.

Transgender people, who identify with a gender that does not correspond to the gender assigned at birth, can identify with the female or male gender, in a binary matrix, or position themselves in any position relative to the gender spectrum.

Non-binary gender identification is often difficult to understand and accept. For most people, the sex assigned to them at birth closely corresponds to their gender identity, as well as the hormones released during puberty and the development of secondary sexual characteristics, making it difficult to understand that for a minority of individuals this may not be the case.

Although in most situations gender is seen as binary, that is, feminine or masculine, over time several non-Western societies have recognized gender outside the binary structure, despite this status not having the corresponding legal recognition. In some cases, a third gender has been recognized. However, this designation does not per se translate into the admission of a gender spectrum. Depending on the legal and social framework, the third gender may correspond to a gender attribution structure that remains rigid but, instead of having two possibilities, has three.

3.3 Non-binary gender in various parts of the world

Although the gender binary has been prevalent and dominant throughout the world for a long time, there have been communities that have recognized gender in a non-binary way, although in most cases it is not about recognizing a gender spectrum, but rather accepting that gender is segmented into fixed categories and that these, instead of two, can be more. Progressively, non-binary gender people have come to have a legal framework for their situation and its consequent recognition in identification documents.

In some communities in Polynesia, people designated as Fa'afafine are considered to be of a third gender.[4] They are anatomically male, but assume a feminine gender expression. In these communities, Fa'afafine people are accepted and recognized as having a non-binary gender.

The Hijra population in India is considered the largest third gender community in the world, with their number estimated at 5 to 6 million individuals. These individuals, classically designated as eunuchs, may be people with DSD or transgender, phenotypically male, wear feminine clothing and identify as being neither men nor women. In her book, Indian photographer Dayanita Singh describes a conversation with a Hijra friend, Mona, in which she asks if Mona would like to have sex reassignment surgery, to which Mona replied "I am not a man who wanted to be a woman, I am a third sex."[5] In 2005, India assumed that there were three possibilities for gender attribution, namely for passports: female, male and eunuch. In 2009, the designation was changed to "others". In 2014, the Supreme Court of India decided that Hijra people could assume the "third gender" and that "transsexual" people could decide their gender identity, opting for the female gender, male gender or third gender.[6]

The Constitutional Court of Nepal approved in 2007 the possibility for identification cards to indicate "third gender" or "other".[7] The same possibility of registration as a third gender exists in Pakistan and Bangladesh.

Thailand has a community of individuals designated as Kathoeys who are usually recognized as being of the third sex. They are people of the male sex at birth, but who identify as having "a feminine heart". Thus, from the point of view of gender expression, they assume feminine representations.

In New Zealand, the designation "indeterminate sex" exists for situations in which it is not possible to determine the sex at the time of birth. In 2012, the designation "X" was included as a possible alternative in the identification documents of people in the process of gender transition.[8] In 2015, a new classification was proposed that includes three possibilities: female, male and gender diverse. In turn, "gender diverse" includes the following subcategories: transgender female to male, transgender male to female and gender diverse not otherwise classified.[9]

In Australia, the gender designation "X" has been possible since 2003. As of 2013, this designation is no longer exclusive to people with indeterminate sex, extending as an option to all adults.[10] In 2019, Tasmania made sex or gender identification optional on birth registration.

In the United States, some states have been implementing, since 2016, the possibility of a non-binary gender "X". This possibility was extended to all citizens in 2022.

In Canada, the way gender is presented on health cards and driver's licenses has been changed. On health cards, gender is no longer mentioned and on driver's licenses it has been possible to designate "X" since 2017. In April 2017, the first person was born with documents that identify a neutral gender "U".[11]

Some indigenous communities in North America recognize more than two genders, with people who are not cisgender male or female being broadly designated as "two spirit".[12,13]

In Europe, in 2015, the European Council issued resolution 2048, towards the recognition of the rights of transgender people. This document expresses that each person should have the right to recognition of their gender identity and the right to be treated and identified according to it. Furthermore, this resolution recommends that each country consider the possibility of including a third gender in the identification documents of those who wish it.[14]

Even before the aforementioned resolution, several countries have adopted non-binary gender designations.

Germany was the first European country, in 2013, to recognize the possibility of non-binary gender, designated as "indeterminate", this being possible for people with DSD with ambiguous genitalia, born from November 2013 onwards. However, in 2015 the legal situation changed, after manifestations of the rights of people with DSD who stated that this designation encouraged sex definition surgeries, it was decided that the gender classification would be female or male but that neither of the two could be assigned. Such an option would be valid not only for new birth registrations of babies with DSD but also for any adult with DSD whose birth registration had been made as male or female. In 2017, the situation was again reviewed by the Federal Constitutional Court, which decided on the existence of a third gender, based on the gender identity of each individual and not on biological sex.

In 2014, Malta introduced the designation "X" as an option for public records and passports. In the same year, Denmark also approved the gender designation "X" in passports.[15] The same thing happened in the Netherlands in 2018 and in Iceland in 2019.

Argentina allowed, from 2012, transgender people to choose the gender they want to have in their identification documents, even without having undergone any gender affirmation treatment. In 2018, it was possible for two transgender people to choose not to have any indication of sex on their identity card. In 2021, a Decree-Law was signed that allows a third gender option, "X", included in the national registry of people (RENAPER), in passports and identity cards.

In Brazil, the situation differs from state to state. In 2022, the State of Rio Grande do Sul allowed non-binary gender people to change their name and gender in the birth registry, according to their gender identity. In Bahia, it became possible to register "non-binary gender" in official documents.

Also in 2022, it became possible to register gender "X" for non-binary gender people in Chile, and "NB" or "no binário" in Colombia.

3.4. Facebook and gender identity

What about Facebook? Although not a country, Facebook is one of the largest communities today. The attribution of gender registration on Facebook varies from country to country, but it has been the subject of discussion and debate in various forums. In the United States, a person who registers on Facebook has 50 gender options available. In the United Kingdom, the available options amount to 71.[16] Despite being considered a marketing strategy, the diversification of gender identities in a community as comprehensive as Facebook can bring positive aspects. First, it allows each person to find a designation with which they identify, then it allows the choice of which pronoun the person prefers to be addressed by, and, above all, it disseminates and makes common different gender designations, facilitating their social acceptance.

3.5. Different gender identities

Gender identification is, in most situations, very early in a child's development. At 2 or 3 years of age, children identify as girls or boys and tend to have different behaviors according to gender.[17] These are the first manifestations of gender expression and identity.

Behaviors such as liking pink clothes with bows and sparkles or enjoying playing with dolls, princess fantasies, or drawing hearts are typically associated with girls, while playing with superheroes, ball games, constructions or toy cars are typically associated with boys.

During the preschool phase, from 3 to 5 years old, and even during elementary school, children react differently to behaviors that violate gender norms. Three more frequent behaviors can be distinguished, which include "correction", "ridicule" and "denial of identity".[18] "Correction" consists of attempts, by other children, to get the child who has a behavior attributable to the opposite gender to modify their actions. For example, they say to a boy, "that doll is for girls, give it to her". "Ridicule" comprises aggressive behaviors that aim at humiliation and try to expose the behavior to ridicule. "Denial of identity" is associated with behaviors in which other children attribute the opposite gender to the child in question. For example, "Sebastian is a girl, he plays with dolls".

However, a fourth type of behavior can be included, which is based on accepting the other as they express themselves. In tolerant family and school environments that support diversity, gender norms and their expression take on less marked contours, which allows children to express themselves more freely and, consequently, more fluidly, being supported by the other children with whom they interact.

The existence of behaviors and expressions attributed as the norm of one gender in a child with sex and gender assigned at birth that does not match that gender is not, by itself, a sign that this child will be transgender. It is important that all children have the possibility to express themselves to their full potential, and school, social and family environments are fundamental pillars for this to happen.

In general, play is encouraged where children can take on all kinds of roles, books with diverse characters that reflect different models, different social roles and different gender identities, sexual orientations and family types.[19,20]

3.5.1. Boys Don't Cry

Manuel was born a boy. He was a perfectly healthy little baby with adequate development. At the age of 3, Manuel ripped off the wallpaper that lined part of his room with spaceships and small dragons with a friendly look that blew smoke out of their noses. I don't like it! I want a castle with princesses, I want fairies with shiny wings and stars!

There was no problem, Manuel's mother changed the wallpaper. White walls appeared with stickers of pink fairies with shiny wings coloring the environment. Manuel loved it. He wanted to be a Fairy.

At school, Manuel was a cheerful boy, he paid a lot of attention to stories, he liked to run, sing and play. But what he liked the most was dressing up as a princess and playing make-believe in the cardboard castle that occupied one of the corners of the room.

At the age of 4, Manuel asked his mother for pink socks with golden stars. The mother agreed and bought the socks. Manuel was super happy. A few days later he took the socks to school. The other boys looked at him, first somewhat shocked, then laughed and started saying: Manuel is a girl! Manuel has pink socks! Manuel ran away and cried. He cried because his friends were making fun of him, he cried because in fact he loved those socks.

Manuel was going to turn 5 and he only wanted one present. He wanted to have a dress. Blue, the color of the sky. The mother didn't know how to face the situation. Until then, she tried to maintain the normality of everyday life and give space and freedom to Manuel for him to play how and with what he wanted, for him to be who he was, and to be happy. But, on that day, on the day that Manuel said he wanted to have a dress, the mother felt that something stronger, more permanent was happening, it was not just a phase.

There was a birthday party, with princesses, elves and fairies and Manuel received his dress. He ran from one side to the other making the blue skirt spin and singing, dancing, with a broad smile.

Days later, one night, before going to sleep, Manuel said to his mother: Mom, you know, I am a girl!

After that day, many others followed, but the speech and behavior did not change. The mother sought information on the subject, spoke with medical and psychology teams, spoke with school teachers and everyone was unanimous that the best strategy would be to allow Manuel to express his inner feeling about who he was. He would be closely monitored in order to detect weaknesses, anxieties and fears, he would be supported in relation to classmates, family and society in general.

Manuel started going to school in dresses, or skirts, pants or shorts, as he wanted. In his room there were drawings of princesses and fairies, dolls, books and colored pencils. Manuel chose a new name and started to be called Violet (the name of his favorite color).

The fictionalized story of Manuel depicts a situation of a child with a gender identity different from the sex and gender assigned at birth. These situations arise in children with totally adequate development and can manifest at different ages, and the manifestations can be very early, at 2 or 3 years of age.

The initial phase usually consists of the manifestation of behaviors and preferences that we attribute as the norm to the opposite gender. Next, the child seeks to express the gender with which they identify and, at this stage, it is typical to seek to express themselves through clothing, haircut, favorite toys, and group of friends. At this stage, hostile behaviors often arise from other children, with situations of mockery, discrimination or distancing. It is essential to have the support of the school so that the child can express themselves and develop freely. The situation must be discussed and explained to the other children, showing that diversity is positive and promoting playful and educational activities with different gender roles and different family models and structures.

Monitoring by health professionals is essential, on the one hand to ensure that the child's physical, mental and social development is adequate, and on the other hand to prevent risk situations associated with these situations.

Later, the child may request other elements in order to identify and be identified with the gender with which they identify. One of the main elements is the name. Although the legal name change does not take place at such early stages, a name with which the child identifies can be chosen and adopted, and they can be treated, at home, at school and, if possible, in all places, by this "new" name. It is up to the parents to explain the situation and ask that the new name be used, especially in situations where the child is called in public, such as at school or in a doctor's waiting room.

The child will grow up and one of the critical points is adolescence. Male adolescents who identify as female do not want to change their voice, have body hair or increase in penis and testicle size. On the other hand, female adolescents who identify as male do not want to have menstruation or breast enlargement. However, this is still a very early age for definitive decisions. But not making a decision can also have definitive consequences.

3.6. Gender expression and affirmation

Gender expression and affirmation is present in each of us and is reflected in the way we make our choices and how we show who we are in terms of practices and behaviors that stem from how we perceive our own gender. Gender expression is part of growth and is present throughout life, manifesting in things as simple as the clothes we wear, our haircut, the sport we dedicate ourselves to, or the car we choose.

When the gender a person identifies with corresponds to the sex and gender assigned to them at birth, gender affirmation, although always present and often very marked, "fits" into social patterns and goes so unnoticed that we don't even think about talking about it.

On the contrary, for people who identify with a gender different from the one designated at birth or for people with a non-binary gender identity, gender affirmation becomes a focal point of development and socially an unavoidable issue, if only because of the difference and what that difference awakens in everyone around them.

As mentioned earlier, gender identity develops very early in child development and, as such, the need to express this very identity, gender expression, also arises at very young ages, such as 2 or 3 years old.

Usually, the first expressions of gender affirmation manifest through the choice of clothing, colors and play activities. It is possible that boys who identify as girls want to wear dresses or skirts, have a preference for pink or other attributes usually associated with the female gender. Girls, in turn, show a preference for pants and shorts and refuse to wear "girl clothes."

In play, boys who identify as girls tend to prefer playing with girls, while girls who identify as boys tend to enjoy playing in groups of boys, showing an appetite for games with a higher level of aggressiveness, soccer games and others traditionally designated as "for boys."

This first level of gender affirmation is relatively discreet since children with a gender identity concordant with the sex and gender assigned at birth also often exhibit this type of preference. Despite everything, in Western societies it is more easily accepted by everyone that a girl has a preference for attributes usually conferred to boys than the reverse situation.

"She's a tomboy." This traditional expression is used to describe girls who like activities, attributes or have behaviors considered typically masculine. This expression does not bring any negative connotation, nor is it directly associated with any type of gender identity or sexual orientation.

On the contrary, popular expressions that designate boys who like activities considered feminine, or have attributes or behaviors considered typically feminine, are connoted with pejorative designations, with discordance in gender identity or homosexuality.

Still at this first level of gender affirmation comes the desire to modify the haircut and hairstyle, an aspect closely associated with the feminine and the masculine.

It is usually around this time that other types of issues with great social impact arise. The child recognizes and often verbalizes that they are (or want to be) of the opposite gender or, less frequently, expresses a non-binary gender identity, saying for example that they are neither a girl nor a boy or that sometimes they are a girl and other times a boy. Furthermore, the child stops identifying with their name and expresses the need to choose a new name, according to the gender they identify with or a gender-neutral name. In addition to the name, the question also arises as to which pronouns should be used (she or he) and how to use all the words that identify them and that have an assigned gender (brother or sister; son or daughter).

These issues are complex due to the diversity of situations they encompass and because they cut across all the contexts in which the child moves, but they are even more complex when the child identifies with a neutral gender and as such would like the language used to also be gender neutral. In the Portuguese language, and in most languages, there are no, for example, gender-neutral personal pronouns in the third person singular (she or he).

At the same time, there are day-to-day practical issues that are of no less importance and deserve reflection. A topic that has been much debated and that, seeming to have a simple solution, is not at all easy, concerns the identification of bathrooms and changing rooms.

In schools, bathrooms are usually divided between boys' bathrooms and girls' bathrooms. How should a child who identifies with a gender different from the sex and gender assigned at birth or who has a non-binary gender identity proceed? The matter is so problematic that some of these children stop going to bathrooms in public places, including at school. This situation leads to serious health problems, both on a psychological level and on a physical level.

At this stage of gender affirmation we have, for example, a child of the female sex who has a male gender identity and who expresses that gender identity by wearing "boy's clothes," including pants, boxers, shirts and typically male sneakers. They have short hair. They play football on the school team and is treated by their colleagues as Jonny (their registered name is Joana). To those looking from the outside, Jonny is a boy. But what if Jonny suddenly enters the girls' bathroom? Or if, in a hospital waiting room, someone calls "Joana" and a young "boy" gets up?

Although the legal name change does not take place in such young children, it is important to find a name with which the child identifies and likes to be called. Often the names chosen by children are gender neutral, and can be given to both female and male people. This name should be used by those around them, at home, at school or in other social contexts. Thus, on the one hand, it is important that parents inform the people involved of the situation and the chosen name, and on the other, it is crucial that institutions, namely schools and health institutions, assume processes of which an active question is part about the gender identity of each person and, in cases of gender identities different from the sex and gender assigned at birth, be asked by what name and pronouns the person wants to be treated. Institutions should also provide inclusive spaces with references (images, posters, books) to all types of people and families, and provide bathrooms, or other types of facilities, that are gender neutral.

If during childhood the physical aspect of the body is not per se very different between boys and girls, the onset of puberty, resulting from the increase in sex hormones, will transform this scenario. It is the phase in which secondary sexual characteristics develop. In girls, menarche, breast development, the appearance of pubic and axillary hair and widening of the pelvis will occur. In boys there will be an increase in muscle mass, a widening of the shoulders, the appearance of hair on the body and face, a widening of the jaw, a deep voice and prominence of the laryngeal cartilage.

For adolescents whose gender identity is different from the sex and gender designated at birth, the appearance of secondary sexual characteristics that identify a gender that they do not recognize as their own is a factor of great anxiety and discomfort, which can be so severe as to motivate self-mutilation, suicidal ideation or even suicide.

At this stage, the recommended strategy is to start puberty-suppressing therapy with gonadotropin-releasing hormone (GnRH) analogues when the adolescent reaches Tanner stage 2 pubertal development (scale for assessing sexual maturation),[21] allowing time to decide on more definitive gender affirmation strategies.[22] It is important that therapy is started early, as some of the secondary sexual characteristics, once developed, are not reversible.

The next step is the use of partially reversible therapies with gender-affirming hormones, estrogens or testosterone. This type of therapy is not usually started before the age of 16, although clinically each case must be considered and evaluated in its own individual way. Starting this type of therapy requires a psychosocial assessment and a thorough clinical assessment to determine possible medical situations in which hormone treatments may be contraindicated.[23] It is necessary to ensure that there is express consent from the individual who will start the treatment and that they are properly informed about its effects and possible adverse effects.

Treatment with estrogens (usually in combination with antiandrogens) will develop female characteristics in individuals who at birth were designated as being male. On the contrary, treatment with testosterone will develop male physical characteristics, namely secondary sexual characteristics, in individuals who at birth were designated as being female, allowing the adolescent to have a physical appearance consistent with the gender with which they identify.

It is important to keep in mind that gender identification is not always binary and the person may not aim for a totally feminine or masculine appearance. Thus, each situation must be analyzed individually, allowing the person to decide on what their goals are in terms of gender identification and expression and on which treatments they do or do not want to do.[24]

3.7. When gender identity does not correspond to the sex assigned at birth - still a medical diagnosis

The most correct designation for situations in which an individual's gender identity is different from the sex and gender assigned at birth is the subject of controversy and discussion.

Over the years, as mentioned in the previous chapter, situations of gender identity that were not congruent with the assigned gender were classified as mental illnesses and treated as pathological. Currently, it is considered that, just as with sexual orientation, different gender identities do not in themselves translate into a disease.

Despite the discussion on the topic, the latest edition of the DSM, DSM-5, classifies this situation as gender dysphoria and establishes the following diagnostic criteria.

Figure 4. Diagnostic criteria for Gender Dysphoria according to DSM-5 - Adapted from DSM-5:

Gender Dysphoria in Children

A. *A marked incongruence between one's experienced/expressed gender and assigned gender, of at least 6 months' duration, as manifested by at least six of the following (one of which must be Criterion A1):*

1. *A strong desire to be of the other gender or an insistence that one is the other gender (or some alternative gender different from one's assigned gender).*

2. *In boys (assigned gender), a strong preference for cross-dressing or simulating female attire; or in girls (assigned gender), a strong preference for wearing only typical masculine clothing and a strong resistance to the wearing of typical feminine clothing.*

3. *A strong preference for cross-gender roles in make-believe play or fantasy play.*

4. *A strong preference for the toys, games, or activities stereotypically used or engaged in by the other gender.*

5. *A strong preference for playmates of the other gender.*

6. *In boys (assigned gender), a strong rejection of typically masculine toys, games, and activities and a strong avoidance of rough-and-tumble play; or in girls (assigned gender), a strong rejection of typically feminine toys, games, and activities.*

7. *A strong dislike of one's sexual anatomy.*

8. *A strong desire for the physical sex characteristics that match one's experienced gender.*

B. The condition is associated with clinically significant distress or impairment in social, occupational, or other important areas of functioning.

Specify if: With a disorder of sex development (DSD)

Gender Dysphoria in Adolescents and Adults

A. A marked incongruence between one's experienced/expressed gender and assigned gender, of at least 6 months' duration, as manifested by at least two of the following:

1. A marked incongruence between one's experienced/expressed gender and primary and/or secondary sex characteristics (or in young adolescents, the anticipated secondary sex characteristics).

2. A strong desire to be rid of one's primary and/or secondary sex characteristics because of a marked incongruence with one's experienced/expressed gender (or in young adolescents, a desire to prevent the development of the anticipated secondary sex characteristics).

3. A strong desire for the primary and/or secondary sex characteristics of the other gender.

4. A strong desire to be of the other gender (or some alternative gender different from one's assigned gender).

5. A strong desire to be treated as the other gender (or some alternative gender different from one's assigned gender).

6. *A strong conviction that one has the typical feelings and reactions of the other gender (or some alternative gender different from one's assigned gender).*

B. The condition is associated with clinically significant distress or impairment in social, occupational, or other important areas of functioning.

Specify if: With Disorder of Sex Development (DSD)

Specify if: Posttransition: The individual has transitioned to full-time living in the desired gender (with or without legalization of gender change) and has undergone (or is preparing to have) at least one cross-sex medical procedure or treatment regimen—namely, regular cross-sex hormone treatment or gender reassignment surgery confirming the desired gender (e.g., penectomy, vaginoplasty in a natal male; mastectomy or phalloplasty in females at birth).

3.8. Prevalence of transgender people

The estimated prevalence of transgender people is difficult, primarily because the definitions of transgender, gender dysphoria, and different gender identities are not consensual and have undergone significant changes over the years.

A systematic review published in 2016[26] evaluated 27 studies on the prevalence of transgender people, assuming the criteria of the authors of the original studies in defining the situation and the study population. Thus, three groups were defined for analysis: prevalence of people who undergo gender-affirming hormone therapies or gender-affirming surgeries; prevalence of people with a diagnosis related to gender identity, applying the different terminologies followed over time by the DSM and ICD; and prevalence of people who define themselves as transgender.

Eight studies were analyzed using the criterion for the prevalence of transgender people that individuals had undergone gender-affirming hormone therapies or gender-affirming surgeries. The studies were published between 1968 and 2014 and conducted in Italy, Spain, Sweden, Netherlands (two), Belgium, United States, and Singapore. The aggregated prevalence was 9.2 per 100,000, 95% CI [4.9-13.6], with a very high heterogeneity between studies. The prevalence of transgender women was 12.5 per 100,000, 95% CI [7.0-17.9] and that of transgender men was 5.1 per 100,000, 95% CI [2.6-7.6].

Regarding the estimated prevalence from studies that used the criterion of people with diagnoses related to gender identity, applying the different terminologies followed over time by the DSM and ICD, 15 studies were analyzed, published between 1968 and 2014, conducted in Spain (two), England and Wales, Scotland, Ireland, Iceland, Sweden, Northern Ireland, Iran, Japan (two), Thailand, United States (two), and Australia. The aggregated prevalence was 6.8 per 100,000, 95% CI [4.6-9.1], also registering a very high heterogeneity between studies. The prevalence of transgender women was 5.8 per 100,000, 95% CI [3.5-8.1] and that of transgender men was 2.5 per 100,000, 95% CI [1.9-3.1].

Finally, the analysis of the prevalence of people who identify as transgender was assessed in six studies, published between 2010 and 2015 and conducted in the Netherlands, Belgium, United States (two), and Taiwan. The aggregate prevalence was 871.2 per 100,000 (0.87%), 95% CI [518.9-1,223.5], again registering a high heterogeneity between studies. The prevalence of transgender women was 846.2 per 100,000 (0.85%), 95% CI [316.5-1,375.9] and that of transgender men was 1,557.5 (1.6%) per 100,000, 95% CI [672.5-2,442.4].

Some studies published after this systematic review and meta-analysis show the following results:

A meta-analysis published in 2017[27] that evaluated the prevalence of people who identify as transgender in the United States included studies from 2007 to 2016, estimating prevalence values of 390 per 100,000 (0.39%), 95% CI [160-620]. However, the most recent study included, the 2016 NCHA data,[28] points to values of 1,790 per 100,000 (1.79%), 95% CI [1,700-1,870]. An analysis of the prevalences of the 13 included studies shows a clear increase in prevalence values in more recent studies. The 2017 NCHA data,[29] not included in the previous meta-analysis, indicate a prevalence of 1.3%.

A narrative review published in 2019, which included 43 studies published between 1968 and 2018, 22 conducted in Europe, 12 in the United States, and the remaining in other countries in Asia, the Middle East, and Australia, points to values of individuals who identify as transgender or non-binary gender between 0.1% and 2% of the population, depending on the country and the criterion used in the classification.[30]

Bibliography

[1] Money J. The concept of gender identity disorder in childhood and adolescence after 39

years. Journal of sex & marital therapy. 1994 Sep 1; 20(3): 163-77.

[2] Money J. Hermaphroditism, gender and precocity in hyperadrenocorticism: psychologic findings. Bulletin of the Johns Hopkins Hospital. 1955 Jun; 96(6): 253-64

[3] Money J., Hampson J. G., Hampson J. L. An examination of some basic sexual concepts: the evidence of human hermaphroditism. Bulletin of the Johns Hopkins Hospital. 1955 Oct; 97(4): 301-19.

[4] Vasey P. L., Bartlett N. H. What can the Samoan «fa'afafine» teach us about the Western concept of gender identity disorder in childhood? Perspectives in biology and medicine. 2007; 50(4): 481-90.

[5] It's Her Story. The Hindu. 3 Feb 2002. http://www.thehindu.com/thehindu/mag/2002/02//03/stories/2002020300230400.htm [Accessed in 4/4/18].

[6] Supreme Court recognizes transgenders as 'third gender'. The Times of India. https://timesofindia.indiatimes.com/india/Supreme-Court-recognizes-transgenders-as-third-gender/ /articleshow/33767900.cms [Accessed in 4/4/18].

[7] Sunil Babu Pant and Others/ v. Nepal Government and Others, Supreme Court of Nepal (21 December 2007). https://www.icj.org/sogicasebook/sunil-babu-pant-and-others-v-nepalgovernment-and-others-supreme-court-of-nepal-21-december-2007/ [Accessed in 4/4/18].

[8] Veale J. F. Prevalence of transsexualism among New Zealand passport holders. Australian & New Zealand Journal of Psychiatry. 2008 Oct; 42(10): 887-9.

[9] Tumanishvili G. G. Universal System Of Sex/Gender Registration. Journal of Law, n.° 2, 2016. http://openjournals.gela.org.ge/index.php/JLow/article/viewFile/1867/1310 . [Accessed in 4/4/18].

[10] Australian Government Guidelines on the Recognition of Sex and Gender. https://www.ag.gov.au//Publications/Pages/AustralianGovernmentGuidelin esontheRecognitionofSexandGender.aspx [Accessed in 4/4/18].

[11] Canadian baby 'first without gender designation' on health card. http://www.bbc.com//news/world-us-canada-40480386 [Accessed in 4/4/18].

[12] Wilson A. How we find ourselves: Identity development and two spirit people. Harvard Educational Review. 1996 Jul 1; 66(2): 303-18.

[13] Hunt S. An introduction to the health of two-spirit people: Historical, contemporary and emergent issues. Prince George, British Columbia, Canada: National Collaborating Centre for Aboriginal Health; 2016.

[14] Discrimination against transgender people in Europe. http://assembly.coe.int/nw/xml/XRef//Xref-XML2HTML-EN.asp?fileid=21736 [Accessed in 2/4/18].

[15] Denmark: X in Passports and New Trans Law Works. https://tgeu.org/denmark-x-in-passportsand-new-trans-law-work/ [Accessed in 2/4/18].

[16] Facebook's 71 gender options come to UK users. https://www.telegraph.co.uk/technology//facebook/10930654/Facebooks-71-gender-options-come-to-UK-users.html [Accessed in 4/4/18].

[17] Martin C. L., Ruble D. N. Patterns of gender development. Annual review of psychology.2010 Jan 10; 61: 353-81.

[18] Martin C. L., Ruble D. N. Patterns of gender development. Annual review of psychology.2010 Jan 10; 61: 353-81.

[19] Healthy Gender Development and Young Children A Guide for Early Childhood Programs and Professionals. https://depts.washington.edu/dbpeds/healthy-gender-development.pdf [Accessed in 4/4/18].

[20] American Psychological Association & National Association of School Psychologists. Resolution on gender and sexual orientation diversity in children and adolescents in schools. 2015.

[21] Tanner J. M. Growth and maturation during adolescence. Nutr Rev. 1981; 39(2): 43-55.

[22] de Vries A. L. C., Steensma T. D., Doreleijers T. A. H., and Cohen-Kettenis P.T. Puberty suppression in adolescents with gender identity disorder: A prospective follow-up study. J Sex Med. 2011; 8: 2276-2283.

[23] Clinical Commissioning Policy: Prescribing of Cross-Sex Hormones as part of the Gender Identity Development Service for Children and Adolescents. August 2016. Published by NHS England.

[24] De Vries A. L. C., Cohen-Kettenis P. T., Delemarre-van de Waal H. A. Clinical management of gender dysphoria in adolescents. Int J Transgenderism. 2007; 9(3): 83-94.

[25] https://www.psychiatry.org/File%20Library/Psychiatrists/Practice/DSM/DSM-5-TR/APA--DSM5TR-GenderDysphoria.pdf [Accessed in 15/11/22].

[26] Collin L., Reisner S. L., Tangpricha V., Goodman M. Prevalence of transgender depends onthe «case» definition: a systematic review. The journal of sexual medicine. 2016 Apr 1; 13(4):613-26.

[27] Meerwijk E. L., Sevelius J. M. Transgender population size in the United States: A metaregression of population-based probability samples. American journal of public health. 2017 Feb; 107(2): e1-8.

[28] American College Health Association. National College Health Assessment. Spring 2016 reference group data report. 2016. http://www.acha-ncha.org/docs/NCHA-II%20SPRING% 202016%20US%20REFERENCE%20GROUP%20DATA%20REPORT.pdf [Accessed in 10/4/18].

[29] American College Health Association. National College Health Assessment. Spring 2017 reference group data report. 2017. http://www.acha-ncha.org/docs/NCHA-II_SPRING_ 2017_REFERENCE_GROUP_DATA_REPORT.pdf [Accessed in 10/4/18].

[30] Goodman, M., Adams, N., Corneil, T., Kreukels, B., Motmans, J., & Coleman, E. (2019). Size and Distribution of Transgender and Gender Nonconforming Populations: A Narrative Review. Endocrinology and metabolism clinics of North America, 48(2), 303-321. https:///doi.org/10.1016/j.ecl.2019.01.001.

Chapter 4 - Will we ever stop being heteronormative?

4.1. Heteronormativity is everywhere

What are we talking about when we talk about heteronormativity? Heteronormativity is present in various aspects of everyday life,[1] such as cinematic representations, books, children's stories, music, advertising, or in everyday conversations. Heteronormativity is everywhere, it is in our individual and collective imagination, in social institutions, health institutions,[2] educational and knowledge systems, work environments or cultural practices.[3]

Expanding this concept, we can say that heteronormative patterns transcend sexual orientation and are also cisnormative since they include gender identity (cisgender) and the binary definition of gender, even in societies that assume themselves as tolerant and open to diversity, both in social and legal terms.

This heteronormative model is transversal to society and imposes itself particularly on children, creating an also heteronormative imaginary. From the outset, this normalization has two direct consequences, on the one hand it alienates, discriminates and often stigmatizes all those who do not fit into this norm and, on the other hand, by reproducing patterns of normativity that are not very comprehensive, it requires that each person makes an effort to face as "normal" something that in fact was not incorporated as such in their daily experience, since childhood.

Heteronormativity assumes a vision of the world in which there are classic patterns of feminine and masculine and where the reference sexual orientation is heterosexual, with the relationship and treatment of homosexual people adapted from what is assumed for heterosexual people. For example, when we evaluate a person, we assume that they are heterosexual "until proven otherwise". When we play with a child or young person, we ask "so do you already have a girlfriend?" (if we are talking to a boy) and "so, do you already have a boyfriend?" (if we are talking to a girl). If we go on the street and see a child dressed in pink or with a doll, we assume that it is a girl, but if they have short hair or a superhero cape, we immediately think that it is a boy. We look at a woman, a man and a child and imagine parents and son or daughter, we look at two women (or two men) and a child and assume it is an uncle, an aunt, a friend.

Moreover, if we assume that a man is heterosexual when in reality he is homosexual we think that "it is normal, we could not know", but if on the contrary we assume that a man is homosexual and he is heterosexual, we are embarrassed, almost wanting to "apologize".[4]

In liberal and tolerant societies, in which legislation imposes equal rights for homosexual and heterosexual people and, in which one tries to give an adequate answer in the sense of gender identity, the existence of a heteronormative pattern constitutes a strong conditioning factor for people, especially children and young people, to assume their identity and become aware of the difference with "normality".[5]

4.2. Heteronormativity in the medical approach

In general, health professionals and medical students assume that they have little or no preparation regarding the approach in a clinical context of sexual orientation and issues related to gender identity. Thus, it is not surprising that in daily clinical practice a hetero and cisnormative approach persists.

In all contexts this approach has negative consequences but, in the clinical context it takes on particular aspects and conditions in an important way the success of the therapeutic relationship and the care provided to patients/people.

By not feeling comfortable with realities that are so often distant to them, health professionals tend to take refuge in known universes and reproduce heteronormative patterns, which with homosexual people or with different gender identities tends to create a communication gap. Moreover, the difficulty in communication is often perceived by people as homophobic, intolerant or discriminatory, when in reality it may only reflect lack of knowledge.

One of the issues that tends to arouse extreme vulnerability on the part of people is non-verbal language, looks, grimaces, physical contact and body posture on the part of the health professional. It is important to consider that most sick people who identify as LGBTQIA+ have already experienced discrimination and anticipate it, which makes them more vulnerable and more sensitive to potential social rejection.[4]

An important aspect that contributes to this situation of unease on the part of health professionals is related to the type of training that is carried out. Most clinical cases presented to students of medicine, nursing or other courses in the health area are governed by heteronormativity and assume traditional roles with regard to gender identity and expression. For example, we may see a clinical case about pregnancy, in which a couple, Inês and Joaquim, is presented, but we will hardly see the same clinical case presented with the couple consisting of Isabel and Joana. If we present a case of a child and say that they live in a normal nuclear family, we immediately assume that they will have a mother and a father, but could they not have two mothers, two fathers, a single mother or a single father, or another type of family structure? Will that be considered a "non-normal" family?

The question arises as to how we understand normality in these contexts. If we understand normality as a statistical distribution, then frequency predominates and some family structures are more common than others. But the normality we are talking about is in the social or even clinical sense and here normality is opposed to abnormality or pathology.

It is fundamental to deconstruct the hegemonic notion that normality is associated with heterosexuality, families with a father and a mother or cisgender people.

The fact that we move in a hetero and cisnormative society creates important inequalities for people who feel excluded from this "normality". In the clinical context, the issue is all the more important as it can condition the degree of exposure and trust of sick people before health professionals, which ultimately distances us from people-centered health and places us in a situation of non-compliance with the principle of equity. In this context, there were several publications by international organizations in order to create more equal health systems and institutions in view of the diversity of people who resort to them.

In 2015, the American College Health Association published guidelines to promote college health programs that are trans-inclusive, providing specific guidance on how to increase tolerance, promote inclusion, and more equitable health care.[6]

In 2011, the Joint Commission International published a document entitled Advancing Effective Communication, Cultural Competence, and Patient- and Family-Centered Care for the Lesbian, Gay, Bisexual, and Transgender (LGBT) Community,[7] defining the need for health institutions and professionals to provide high quality health services, respecting the diversity of people, in an individual-centered practice. This document places special emphasis on professional communication between doctor and sick person, on the empathetic and trusting relationship.

In 2014, the Association of American Medical Colleges published a document entitled Implementing Curricular and Institutional Climate Changes to Improve Health Care for Individuals Who Are LGBT, Gender Nonconforming, or Born with DSD[8] which is based on the assumption that medical students have little or no information about the LGBTQIA+ population in their academic curriculum, which constitutes a huge barrier to the future relationship with LGBTQIA+ people, making it urgent to incorporate this theme, in all its diversity, into academic curricula. The document reflects, among other themes, on health disparities, on communication and on specific health needs of the LGBTQIA+ population.

The American Medical Association provides on its website several contents that aim to promote an inclusive medical practice that addresses the diversity of gender identities and sexual orientations.[9]

In 2017, the European Commission published a report entitled State-of-the-art study focusing on the health inequalities faced by LGBTI people,[10] within the scope of the Health4LGBTI project, which analyzes and reflects on health inequalities of the LGBTI population in the European Union, and the impact this has on their health.

In 2019, the Directorate-General for Health published the Health Strategy for Lesbian, Gay, Bisexual, Trans and Intersex people – LGBTI, with Volume 1 dedicated to responding to the health needs of transgender and intersex people, particularly with regard to clinical monitoring and possible medical and surgical procedures. The definition of a strategy for action and planning of targeted and personalized care is essential to establish a path towards equality and equity.[11]

In 2020, the European Commission report, Union of Equality: Strategy for Equal Treatment of LGBTQ+ People, 2020-2025, reinforces the idea that there is huge inequality in health care and in the health of people belonging to sexual and/or gender minorities, with special emphasis on the need to find strategies to reduce this gap.[12]

Although inclusion and respect for diversity must be present in each and every clinical act, there are some situations that, due to their frequency, importance or vulnerability, deserve to be highlighted, among others, the topics described below, which will be detailed in other chapters:

- Communication with adolescents and adults about sexual orientation.
- Communication with children and adolescents about gender identity.
- Communication with adults about sexual practices.
- Prenatal, during childbirth and postnatal communication with lesbian families.[13]
- Communication with children and parents in lesbian or gay families.
- Communication and assessment of lesbian or gay people who individually or as a couple intend to have children.

- Communication and assessment of transgender people.
- Communication and assessment of people with different sexual development (DSD).
- Management and communication of visitors and companions in the context of health care for LGBTQIA+ people.
- Communication with LGBTQIA+ older people.

Bibliography

[1] Herz M., Johansson T. The normativity of the concept of heteronormativity. Journal of Homosexuality. 2015 Aug 3; 62(8): 1009-20.

[2] Röndahl G. Heteronormativity in a nursing context: attitudes toward homosexuality and experiences of lesbians and gay men (Doctoral dissertation, Acta Universitatis Upsaliensis). Accessed in http://www.diva-portal.org/smash/record.jsf?pid=diva2%3A166121&dswid=5196 [Accessed in 30/3/2018].

[3] Yep G. A. The violence of heteronormativity in communication studies: Notes on injury, healing, and queer world-making. Journal of homosexuality. 2003 Sep 23; 45(2-4): 11-59.

[4] Wilton T. Sexualities in health and social care. Sexualities in health and social care. Buckingham: Open University Press. 2000 Jul. p22.

[5] Platzer H., James T. Lesbians' experiences of healthcare. NT Research. 2000 May; 5(3): 194-202.

[6] American College Health Association. ACHA Guidelines for trans-inclusive college health programs. Hanover, Maryland: www. acha. org. 2015. [Accessed in 30/3/2018]

[7] The Joint Commission: Advancing Effective Communication, Cultural Competence, and Patientand Family- Centered Care for the Lesbian, Gay, Bisexual, and Trans- gender (LGBT) Community: A Field Guide. Oak Brook, IL, Oct. 2011.

[8] Hollenbach A. D., Eckstrand K. L., Dreger A. D., editors. Implementing curricular and institutional climate changes to improve health care for individuals who are LGBT, gender nonconforming, or born with DSD: a resource for medical educators. Association of American Medical Colleges; 2014.

[9] https://www.ama-assn.org/delivering-care/physician-resources-lgbtq-inclusive-practice [Acesso em 1/4/2018].

[10] Zeeman L., Sherriff N., Browne K., McGlynn N., Aujean S., et al. TASK 1: State-of-the-art study focusing on the health inequalities faced by LGBTI people D1.1 State-of-the-Art Synthesis Report (SSR). ec.europa.eu/health/social_determinants/projects/ep_funded_projects_en.htm#fragment2. [Accessed in 30/4/18].

[11] Estratégia de saúde para as pessoas lésbicas, gays, bissexuais, trans e intersexo. Lisboa: Ministério da Saúde. Direção-Geral da Saúde. 2019.

[12] União Europeia. União da Igualdade: Estratégia para a igualdade de tratamento das pessoas LGBTIQ 2020-2025 [Internet]. União Europeia. 2020. Available from: https://eurlex. europa.eu/legal-content/PT/TXT/?uri=CELEX%3A52020DC0698 [Accessed in 4/10/22].

[13] Röndahl G., Bruhner E., Lindhe J. Heteronormative communication with lesbian families in antenatal care, childbirth and postnatal care. Journal of Advanced Nursing. 2009 Nov 1;65(11): 2337-44.

Ana Macedo

Chapter 5 - **Differences in Sexual Development (DSD)**

5.1. Nomenclature and classifications of differences in sexual development (DSD)

Differences in sexual development (DSD) have been the subject of discussion and targeted by many definitions over time. Currently, they are defined as congenital situations in which the chromosomal, gonadal, or anatomical development of the sexual organs is atypical.

The nomenclature associated with these situations is controversial and has been changing over the years, either due to the advancement of knowledge in this matter or in response to ethical and social issues.[1,2] The designation DSD was adopted as a result of the Chicago Consensus Meeting in 2005 and succeeded the previously used terminology that referred to these situations as intersex.[3,4]

The classic nomenclature of situations with atypical sexual development was based on the texts of Theodor Albrecht Edwin Klebs, published in 1876.

Klebs, a German-Swiss pathologist who lived between 1834 and 1913, developed his work mainly in the study of infectious diseases, having been one of the inspirers of the later works of Louis Pasteur and Robert Koch. In an era prior to modern genetics, Klebs was responsible for a classification of the so-called hermaphrodites according to the nature of the gonads, subdividing them into three types: male pseudo-hermaphrodites (ambiguous genitalia with testicles), female pseudo-hermaphrodites (ambiguous genitalia with ovaries), and true hermaphrodites if they simultaneously presented at least one ovary and one testicle.[5]

The classification model proposed by Klebs was incorporated into medical practice from the beginning of the 20th century. This model made the notion prevail that the "true sex" depends on the gonads (ovary and testicle). However, in 1915, William Bell questioned this definition, giving as an example a case of an individual with androgen insensitivity syndrome who, having testicles, presented an entirely feminine physical appearance, given the absence of cellular response to testosterone. Bell assumed that the "true sex" should not be determined by non-functioning ovaries or testicles to the detriment of the entire physical development.

Only many years later, with the advancement of knowledge in the field of genetics, were the classic classifications redefined, and the terminology of genital ambiguity with 46, XY karyotype or genital ambiguity with 46, XX karyotype began to be used.

The Chicago Consensus Meeting[3] brought significant changes to the terminology used, considering that the nomenclature associated with any situation should always take into account the sensitivities of the sick people, be sufficiently flexible to accommodate new information that emerges, and, at the same time, be scientifically robust and consistent.

In this context, it is understood that one should seek to find terms that describe the genetic etiology and, at the same time, include phenotypic variations. Despite advances in molecular genetics having revealed some of the underlying causes of some DSD, a specific molecular diagnosis is only possible in about 20% of cases.[6]

Terms such as hermaphroditism, pseudohermaphroditism, sex reversal, and intersex, after being the target of controversy and contestation, were considered to be scientifically imprecise and socially pejorative.[7]

The following tables reflect the nomenclature proposed by the Chicago Consensus Meeting. Despite the advances brought by the Chicago Consensus Meeting, unresolved issues and disagreements continued to exist. In 2016, an update of the consensus was published,[8] which was subscribed by the European Society for Pediatric Endocrinology, Pediatric Endocrine Society, Australian Pediatric Endocrine Group, Asian Pacific Pediatric Endocrine Society, Japanese Society of Pediatric Endocrinology, Sociedad Latino-Americana de Endocrinologia Pediatrica, and the Chinese Society of Pediatric Endocrinology and Metabolism.

In this update, the various stakeholders consider that although the term DSD has been accepted by most health professionals, this terminology has not been universally accepted by sick people and support groups for patients and families.[9] In the re-analysis of the Chicago consensus, the most positive aspects that stand out are the existence of a scientifically valid term in the medical and biological context and the existence of a classification system that can be integrated into health models and that differentiates itself from other situations of gender identity or sexual orientation. On the other hand, the stigma associated with the term "disorder" and the fact that the word "sexual" can be understood as sexual behavior have been reported as negative aspects. Furthermore, the designation may not be fully applicable to certain individuals, such as men with congenital adrenal hyperplasia.

The proposals are in the sense of being able to replace the word "disorders" with "differences," maintaining the term intersex, or finding another alternative nomenclature.

5.2. Incidence of DSD

The different designations and the use of often not very consensual terminology have contributed to the difficulty of estimating the incidence of individuals who are born with differences in sexual development and with genital ambiguity.[10] The data point to values of approximately 1 in 4,500 to 5,000.[11]

The incidence of DSD in 46, XY individuals was estimated at 1 in 20,000 live births, while the incidence of DSD in 46, XX individuals, mostly in the context of congenital adrenal hyperplasia (CAH), was estimated at 1 in 14,000-15,000 live births.[12]

The incidence of ovotesticular DSD was estimated at 1 in 100,000 live births[13] and that of testicular or mixed gonadal dysgenesis at 1 in 10,000.[14]

It is estimated that mixed gonadal dysgenesis and CAH together represent about half of all DSD in which individuals present with ambiguous genitalia.[15]

5.3. Evaluation of a person with genital ambiguity

The evaluation of a child with ambiguous genitalia or atypical genitalia is based primarily on clinical history and physical examination, and the evaluation should be carried out by a multidisciplinary team, aiming at a definitive diagnosis.[16,17]

The identification of a DSD situation can occur early, but it can also be detected later, during childhood, adolescence, or even in adult life. Early presentation forms are often detected in the first observation of the newborn in which it is verified that the newborn presents with ambiguous genitalia, whose appearance is discordant with the karyotype or prenatal ultrasound evaluation. Late presentations are variable and may include situations such as phenotypically male individuals who have cyclic hematuria, phenotypically female individuals who present progressive virilization during puberty, delayed pubertal development, or incomplete development.

In all situations, it is essential to obtain as much detail as possible about the prenatal history and family history, in order to identify possible congenital diseases.

The existence of a prenatal karyotype allows the detection of chromosomal mosaicisms and/or discrepancies between the chromosomal sex and the phenotype, both evaluated by prenatal ultrasound and by physical examination after birth.

In addition to history taking, the physical examination should include a careful evaluation of the external genitalia, including the presence of palpable gonads and evaluation of asymmetries.

Imaging evaluation should be appropriate for each situation but may include imaging exams of the pelvis and abdomen. Laboratory evaluation is specific for each situation. In case of suspected CAH, it includes 17-hydroxyprogesterone, androstenedione, deoxycortisol, renin, ACTH, and electrolyte panel.

Until relatively recently, the dominant idea was that there would be a benefit in making a gender definition (redefinition) as early as possible through surgery and/or hormonal treatments.[4] Currently, it is controversial whether one should intervene, potentially irreversibly, in a gender assignment in babies or children, since they cannot express their will or feelings.

Gender identity has been studied in some groups of people who were born with DSD. The results show that there is no homogeneous pattern. According to recommendations published in 2006, individuals with 46, XX CAH should be "assigned" a female gender, since it was estimated that 90%

would identify with the female gender in adolescence and adult life.[18] Similarly, it was considered that 46, XY individuals with complete androgen insensitivity syndrome (CAIS) should be considered as female gender,[19] with the respective reconstruction of the genitals, since the majority of these would identify in adult life as being of female gender. However, in a situation of PAIS (partial insensitivity), it is estimated that about 25% of individuals may not identify with the gender assigned to them.[20]

Regarding babies born with 5-reductase deficiency or 17-hydroxysteroid dehydrogenase-3 deficiency, the recommendations were less clear since more than half of the individuals who were treated as female did not identify with this gender.[21]

Despite the limited evidence available on the topic, surgeries for redefining sexual organs have been a common practice in cases of newborns or children with DSD. Surgeries performed on people with DSD and ambiguous genitalia may include vaginoplasty, labioplasty, phalloplasty, and gonadal removal. In these situations, the surgery is not performed based on the karyotype, but rather on the diagnosis, anatomical characteristics, hormonal values, and fertility potential.

One of the main reasons cited for performing early surgeries is the reduction of family stress and anxiety levels.[22] It is not easy to manage the proper growth and development of a child who presents a different sexual development. However, increasingly, the recommendations are to postpone any redefinition of sexual organs until the child has a defined gender identity and can express their will and consent, except when there is a health risk.

Bibliography

[1] Frader J., Alderson P., Asch A., et al. Health care professionals and intersex conditions. Arch Pediatr Adolesc Med. 2004; 158: 426-9

[2] Dreger A. D., Chase C., Sousa A., et al. Changing the nomenclature/taxonomy for intersex: A scientific and clinical rationale. J Pediatr Endocrinol Metab. 2005; 18: 729-33.

[3] Hughes I. A., Houk C., Ahmed S. F., Lee P. A. Consensus statement on management of intersex disorders. Journal of pediatric urology. 2006 Jun 1; 2(3): 148-62.

[4] Lee P. A., Houk C. P., Ahmed S. F., Hughes I. A. Consensus statement on management of intersex disorders. Pediatrics. 2006 Aug 1; 118(2): e488-500.

[5] Holmes, Morgan, eds. Critical Intersex. Farnham, England: Ashgate, 2009. P.81

[6] Ono M., Harley V. R. Disorders of sex development: new genes, new concepts. Nat Rev Endocrinol. 2013 Feb; 9(2): 79-91.

[7] Conn J., Gillam L., Conway G. Revealing the diagnosis of androgen insensitivity syndrome in adulthood. BMJ. 2005; 331: 628-30

[8] Lee P. A., Nordenström A., Houk C. P., Ahmed S. F., Auchus R., Baratz A., Dalke K. B., Liao L. M., Lin-Su K., Looijenga 3rd L. H., Mazur T. Global disorders of sex development update since 2006: perceptions, approach and care. Hormone research in paediatrics. 2016; 85(3): 158-80.

[9] Pasterski V., Prentice P., Hughes I. A.: Consequences of the Chicago consensus on disorders of sex development (DSD): current practices in Europe. Arch Dis Child. 2010; 95: 618-623.

[10] Blackless M., Charuvastra A., Derryck A., Fausto-Sterling A., Lauzanne K., Lee E: How sexually dimorphic are we? Review and synthesis. Am J Hum Biol. 2000; 12: 151-166.

[11] Sax L: How common is intersex? A response to Anne Fausto-Sterling. J Sex Res. 2002; 39: 174-178.

[12] Pang S. Y., Wallace M. A., Hofman L., Thuline H. C., Dorche C., Lyon I. C., Dobbins R. H., Kling S., Fujieda K., Suwa S: Worldwide experience in newborn screening for classical. congenital adrenal hyperplasia due to 21-hydroxylase deficiency. Pediatrics. 1988; 81:

866-874.

[13] Nistal M., Paniagua R., Gonzalez-Peramato P., Reyes-Mugica M: Ovotesticular DSD (true hermaphroditism). Pediatr Dev Pathol. 2015; 18: 345-352.

[14] Skakkebaek N. E., Rajpert-De Meyts E., Main K. M.: Testicular dysgenesis syndrome: an increasingly common developmental disorder with environmental aspects. Hum Reprod. 2001; 16: 972-978.

[15] Thyen U., Lanz K., Holterhus P. M., Hiort O: Epidemiology and initial management of ambiguous genitalia at birth in Germany. Horm Res. 2006; 66: 195-203.

[16] Ahmed S. F., Achermann J. C., Arlt W., Balen A. H., Conway G., Edwards Z. L., Elford S., Hughes I. A., Izatt L., Krone N., Miles H. L., O'Toole S., Perry L., Sanders C., Simmonds M., Wallace A. M., Watt A., Willis D: UK guidance on the initial evaluation of an infant or an adolescent with a suspected disorder of sex development. Clin Endocrinol (Oxf) 2011; 75: 12-26.

[17] Adam M. P., Fechner P. Y., Ramsdell L. A., Badaru A., Grady R. E., Pagon R. A., McCauley E., Cheng E. Y., Parisi M. A., Shnorhavorian M: Ambiguous genitalia: what genetic testing is practical? Am J Med Genet A. 2012; 158A: 1337-1343.

[18] Dessens A. B., Slijper F. M., Drop S. L. Gender dysphoria and gender change in chromosomal females with congenital adrenal hyperplasia. Archives of sexual behavior. 2005 Aug 1; 34(4): 389-97.

[19] Mazur T. Gender dysphoria and gender change in androgen insensitivity or micropenis. Archives of Sexual Behavior. 2005 Aug 1; 34(4): 411-21.

[20] Krishna K. B., Houk C. P., Lee P. A. Pragmatic approach to intersex, including genital ambiguity, in the newborn. InSeminars in perinatology. 2017 Jun 1 (Vol. 41, No. 4, pp. 244-251).

[21] Cohen-Kettenis P. T. Gender change in 46, XY persons with 5α-reductase-2 deficiency and 17β-hydroxysteroid dehydrogenase-3 deficiency. Archives of Sexual Behavior. 2005 Aug 1; 34(4): 399-410.

[22] Lee P. A., Wisniewski A. B., Baskin L., Vogiatzi M. G., Vilain E., Rosenthal S. M., Houk C. Advances in diagnosis and care of persons with DSD over the last decade. International Journal of Pediatric Endocrinology. 2014 Dec; 2014(1): 19.

Chapter 6. Hormonal and surgical treatment for gender affirmation

6.1. Hormonal treatment for gender affirmation

Hormonal treatment for gender affirmation can be subdivided into two groups: treatments aimed at preventing pubertal development and those that include the direct administration of female or male hormones, seeking a physical and psychological modification in the feminine or masculine direction.

Regarding treatments aimed at preventing pubertal development, gonadotropin-releasing hormone (GnRH) analogs are used. These are reversible, meaning their effect disappears after discontinuation, allowing the pubertal development to start or continue, and they do not imply a binary structuring, meaning they do not seek to develop feminine or masculine characteristics, but rather to avoid the sexualization of the body that occurs in adolescence. These treatments allow time to be gained for a future decision, reflected upon and matured by the child/youth in their family and social context.

The onset of puberty in a child with a gender identity different from the sex assigned at birth raises very problematic and disruptive issues, as adolescence brings with it the accentuation of characteristics with which the child does not identify and makes them visible to "the world".

Treatments with female or male hormones, estrogens and antiandrogens or testosterone, have some reversible effects, but others are irreversible. In people with a gender identity different from the sex assigned at birth but with a binary gender identity, these treatments are applied aiming to obtain the secondary sexual characteristics of the gender with which the person identifies. In other words, the goal is to suppress the hormones that the body would produce endogenously according to its biological sex and to administer exogenously the hormones corresponding to the gender with which the person identifies (which in a binary structure corresponds to the opposite sex).

In people with a non-binary gender identity, hormonal treatments for gender affirmation (or gender affirmation surgeries) pose other challenges. It is important to understand and explain to each person considering the possibility of starting a treatment what the effect of the treatment will be, that is, what will change in the body, including in the psychic sphere. On the other hand, it is crucial to explicitly ask about the goals of the person in question.

Expectations, especially in people whose gender identity is non-binary, may not be simple to define. For the success of the chosen options, it is essential to make a correct assessment of these expectations and align them according to the existing therapeutic alternatives.

It is important to consider that an individual can be transgender without having undergone or wanting to undergo any type of surgery or hormonal therapy.

As mentioned earlier, the transformation process of a transgender individual occurs in several sequential phases, some reversible and others irreversible, and depends on the individual's desire for change and how they express their gender identity, especially regarding the physical aspect with which they identify.

The first phase of the transformation process and of approximation to the typical aesthetic and behavioral models for the gender with which the person identifies usually involves changes in clothing, haircut, behaviors, and activities. Especially in children, these modifications are very relevant, happen at a very early age, and translate into a significant improvement in quality of life and self-image.

6.1.1. Puberty suppression

In a second phase, and considering that it is a child who will eventually enter the pubertal phase, treatment with GnRH analogs is considered. These, by preventing the development of secondary sexual characteristics, will give the child's body a sexually more immature and less differentiated appearance, allowing them to maintain the previously defined aesthetic choices without confronting a sexual identity that does not correspond to the gender with which they identify.

Let's recall the girl who, at 3 or 4 years old, starts refusing to wear dresses and skirts, wants pants, shorts, and soccer cleats. She cuts her hair short and plays on the school team with "the other boys". She asks to be called Jonny and, apart from a few pesky and unpleasant kids, everything is going well. Looking at her, she is "a him", on the street, in stores, in restaurants, they often confuse her. But that's good...

Only Jonny will grow up. At 10, 11 years old, things threaten to start changing. The breasts begin to increase in size, menstruation may appear... At this point, it is common for fear to set in. This fear is important and should not be minimized, as its consequences can be serious. The suicide attempt rate is very high in transgender youth.

Puberty corresponds to an increase in amplitude and frequency of gonadotropin-releasing hormone (GnRH) pulses and consequent stimulation of the gonads. GnRH is released by the hypothalamus and acts on the pituitary gland, which in turn releases luteinizing hormone (LH) and follicle-stimulating hormone (FSH). These act on the gonads (ovaries and testicles), promoting the production of mature gametes and the synthesis of sex steroids, estradiol in the case of women and testosterone in the case of men.[1]

The use of GnRH analogs will inhibit the hypothalamic-pituitary-gonadal axis, limiting the amplitude and frequency of GnRH pulses and having the final consequence of inhibiting the synthesis of estradiol or testosterone. Thus, the hormonal conditions of childhood are maintained without the appearance or development of secondary sexual characteristics. The inhibition of the onset of puberty with GnHR analogs is reversible with the discontinuation of therapy.

6.1.2. Hormonal therapy for female gender affirmation

As the adolescent individual gets older, in most situations, they want their body to change according to the gender with which they identify. In this context, treatment with GnHR analogs and the consequent inhibition of pubertal development are no longer adequate. The next step will be to start treatment with sex hormones.

According to the World Professional Association for Transgender Health (WPATH), the criteria for initiating hormonal treatment for gender affirmation with sex hormones are the diagnosis of gender dysphoria (see below), the ability to give informed consent, the age of majority, and adequate control of significant medical or psychological comorbidities.[2,3]

It is important that this type of treatment is initiated after conscious reflection by the young person, and for this, maturity and time for consideration are necessary, but it is equally important that the treatment is carried out at the right time, avoiding the development of secondary sexual characteristics that will be difficult or impossible to reverse.

In the case of a transgender female (male-to-female transition), treatment should ideally be initiated before there are changes in voice tone, the appearance of laryngeal prominence, growth or appearance of facial hair. These secondary sexual characteristics will not be avoided if the young person starts treatment after puberty is complete or almost complete, even if antiandrogens and estradiol are administered.

Treatment with antiandrogens can be performed with spironolactone, a specific aldosterone agonist and a competitive inhibitor of androgen receptors. The recommended dose is 100 to 400 mg/day.[4]

Another possibility is the administration of cyproterone acetate, which is a progesterone derivative and, at the same time, an androgen receptor inhibitor. The recommended dose is 50 to 100 mg/day.[4,5]

Estrogen treatment is usually performed with estradiol (17-beta estradiol) or conjugated preparations, orally, 2 to 6 mg/day, or transdermal estradiol, 100 to 200 mcg twice a week. Parenteral administration is sometimes used when target values cannot be obtained with oral or transdermal therapy.[5]

Ethinyl estradiol, present in oral contraceptives, has been used in the treatment of transgender women, but its use has been discouraged due to the risk of venous thromboembolism (VTE)[6] and cardiovascular death.[5]

There is no defined age limit up to which estrogen therapy should be maintained in a transgender woman. From the age of 50, its reduction can be considered in people who have undergone gonadectomy, since this is the age at which cisgender women enter menopause.[7]

In transgender women with cardiovascular risk factors or cardiovascular disease, transdermal estrogens should be used due to their lower risk of VTE and potential changes in lipid profile and coagulation. Although the level of available evidence is limited due to the absence of large-scale studies with controlled samples, the work carried out to date suggests that the use of estrogens in transgender women confers an increased risk of myocardial infarction and ischemia. Conversely, there is no evidence that in transgender men receiving testosterone there is an increased risk of cardiovascular or cerebrovascular diseases.[8]

Both the hormones used in transgender women and the hormonal regimens used in transgender men are safe when used within established protocols and are associated with significant improvements in mental health, including a reduction in situations of depression and anxiety.[9]

Clinical Effects

After starting treatment with estrogens in individuals designated as male at birth, the following changes are expected[5,10]:

- Decrease in sexual desire – onset after 1 to 3 months; maximum after 3 to 6 months;
- Decrease in spontaneous erections – onset after 1 to 3 months; maximum after 3 to 6 months;
- Decrease in muscle strength and mass – onset after 3 to 6 months; maximum after 1 to 2 years;

- Increase in mammary glands – onset after 3 to 6 months; maximum after 2 to 3 years;

- Decrease in testicular volume – onset after 3 to 6 months; maximum after 2 to 3 years;

- Increase and redistribution of body fat – onset after 3 to 6 months; maximum after 2 to 3 years;

- The skin becomes softer and less oily – onset after 3 to 6 months;

- Decrease in facial and body hair – onset 6 to 12 months; maximum after more than 3 years;

- Decrease in sperm production – maximum after more than 3 years;

- Decrease in growth – variable.

The time to obtain maximum modification varies from individual to individual but is between 18 and 36 months. The use of adjuvant antiandrogen therapy can enhance the effect obtained.

Antiandrogens and estrogens have no effect on voice tone, so this modification requires speech therapy in a specialized center. The therapy focuses mainly on resonance and voice tone, since the combination of these two characteristics seems to be determinant for the way the gender of the speaker is interpreted.[5,11,12]

Adverse Effects

The main adverse effects related to female gender affirmation hormone treatment include venous thromboembolism (VTE), cardiovascular disease, increased triglycerides, hyperprolactinemia, and risk of breast cancer.[5]

VTE has an incidence of 2% to 6% in the female transgender population treated with oral ethinyl estradiol. However, the evidence of increased risk with administration of 17-beta estradiol was not conclusive, with some studies showing an increase and others presenting a risk similar to that of the general population.[7,13]

VTE is also associated with prolonged surgery, immobilization after surgery, smoking, and hypercoagulability states.[14]

VTE prophylaxis is not generally recommended for all female transgender individuals, having specific indications for situations of increased risk.

Prothrombotic or hypercoagulability states, or a family history of hypercoagulability are considered situations of increased risk, and in these situations, it is recommended to follow the same guidelines as in the general population, namely the use of anticoagulation or antiplatelet therapy. In these contexts, the risk of treatment with estrogens should be considered, and the choice should fall on transdermal estrogens.[7]

In the presence of other risk factors such as tobacco or situations of prolonged immobilization, prophylaxis should be considered according to the guidelines for the general population.[7]

If an episode of VTE occurs in an individual undergoing estrogen therapy, it should be interrupted during the acute episode of VTE. Subsequently, and depending on the probable cause for the VTE episode, the risks of estrogen therapy and the possibility of administering it transdermally, as well as the need for long-term prophylaxis, should be considered.[7]

Elevated prolactin levels and prolactinomas are risks theoretically associated with estrogen therapy. However, there is no clear evidence of an increased risk in transgender women compared to cisgender women in situations where physiological doses of estrogens are administered. The Endocrine Society's recommendations are not to measure prolactin in routine exams but only in situations where there are symptoms such as new-onset headaches, visual changes, or galactorrhea.[7,15,16]

Treatment Monitoring

In transgender women undergoing hormonal therapy, treatment monitoring should be performed every three months during the first year and then once or twice a year, or whenever treatment is modified[5,10,17,18,19]:

- Monitoring of feminization and adverse effects every 3 months in the first year and then every 6 to 12 months, including hematocrit, blood glucose, and lipid profile;
- Monitoring of serum testosterone during the first 6 months until levels are below 55 ng/dL;
- Monitoring of serum estradiol in follow-up evaluations, with target values of 100 to 200 pg/mL. There is no evidence that higher levels of estrogens result in greater feminization;

- Estrogen doses should be adjusted based on serum estradiol levels. It is important to note that conjugated estrogens and ethinyl estradiol are not adequately evaluated by the laboratory techniques commonly used in estrogen dosing, resulting in lower laboratory values.

- Evaluation of bone mineral density in individuals at risk for osteoporosis, or those over 60 years of age or with consistently low sex hormone levels;

- Initial prolactin evaluation, 12 months after starting therapy, and then every 2 years;

- Evaluation of serum electrolytes, especially potassium levels, in individuals receiving spironolactone every 2 or 3 months during the first year of treatment;

- Screening for breast cancer and, if applicable, prostate cancer.

6.1.3. Masculine Gender Affirmation Hormone Therapy

In the case of a transgender male (female-to-male transition), treatment should ideally be initiated before there is a significant increase in the mammary gland. The main goals to be achieved with hormone therapy include amenorrhea and virilization, namely an increase in facial and body hair, an increase in the clitoris, and masculinization of the body through muscle development and modification of the body fat pattern.

Testosterone

Although testosterone exists in various types of preparations and routes of administration, the treatment of choice is the intramuscular administration of testosterone at doses of 50 to 100 mg weekly or 200 mg every two weeks. Compared to topical routes of administration, injectable forms allow for higher serum concentrations.

There is no defined age limit up to which testosterone therapy should be maintained in a transgender man. From the age of 50, a reduction in testosterone can be considered, since this is the age at which cisgender women enter menopause.[7]

Clinical Effect

In transgender male individuals, the following changes are expected after starting treatment with testosterone:[20,21,22]

- Amenorrhea – after 1 to 6 months;
- Clitoral enlargement – onset 1 to 6 months; maximum 1 to 2 years;
- Vaginal atrophy – onset 1 to 6 months; maximum 1 to 2 years;
- Skin changes and acne – onset 1 to 6 months; maximum 1 to 2 years;
- Changes in body fat distribution – onset 1 to 6 months; maximum after 2 to 5 years;
- Increase in body and facial hair – onset 6 to 12 months; maximum after more than 3 years;
- Increase in muscle mass and strength – onset 6 to 12 months; maximum after 2 to 5 years;

- Voice change becoming deeper – onset 6 to 12 months; maximum after 1 to 2 years;
- Increased libido.

Side effects

Testosterone treatment is safe for most individuals.[23] The main adverse effects related to masculinizing gender-affirming hormone treatment include persistent menstruation, erythrocytosis, and changes in lipid profile.[20]

Monitoring

After starting therapy, the monitoring recommendations for transgender men receiving testosterone include[20,24,25,26]:

• Monitoring virilization and adverse effects every 3 months in the first year and then every 6 to 12 months, including hematocrit, lipid profile, liver function, body weight and blood pressure;

• Monitoring serum testosterone at follow-up assessments, with target values of 350 to 700 ng/dL;

• Monitoring serum estradiol during the first 6 months and until amenorrhea. Estradiol values should be below 50 pg/mL;

• Assessment of bone mineral density in individuals at risk for osteoporosis, or those over 60 years or with consistently low sex hormone levels;

• Screening for breast cancer and, if applicable, cervical cancer.

Hormone therapy is associated with an increase in quality of life for transgender people, with positive effects on both mood and sexual function and a reduction in stress levels.[27] In addition to the positive effect associated with gender expression consistent with gender identity, there is evidence that testosterone may have the effect of increasing serotonin reuptake,[28] a neurotransmitter that is reduced in depression situations.

6.2. Female gender affirmation surgeries

Gender affirmation surgery is one of the last phases in the transition process for transgender people. However, this is not a mandatory phase or a phase that all transgender people want to go through. A transgender person may, as previously mentioned, choose not to have any type of surgery or even choose not to have hormone therapy.

The various female gender affirmation surgeries aim, on the one hand, to excise the male sexual organs and, on the other hand, to reconstruct female external sexual organs and feminize the body and face. In the case of transgender women, surgeries include prostatectomy, orchiectomy and genital reconstruction surgeries, vaginoplasty, breast reconstruction and other surgeries that include facial feminization, rhinoplasty, jaw angle reduction, thyroid cartilage reduction, liposuction and buttock implants.

6.2.1. Vaginoplasty

Vaginoplasty consists of the reconstruction of the female external genital structures, including the creation of a vaginal canal. The surgery aims to create a clitoris, a functional female vulva and a vaginal cavity, with labia minora and majora, that allows penetration during sexual intercourse.[29] The goal is for each surgery to have minimal complications and the best aesthetic and functional effect. There are currently several surgical techniques for vaginoplasty, the most frequently used being the so-called penile inversion. As an alternative, the pedicled colon flap technique can be mentioned.[30]

Procedures prior to surgery include long-term or permanent hair removal procedures of the scrotum and perineum area, since in vaginoplasties with penile inversion, local grafts from the penis and scrotum are used, and the possibility of subsequent hair growth should be minimized.[31]

Another important procedure is thromboprophylaxis. In the female transgender population, there are several factors that contribute to an increased incidence of thromboembolic events, namely the administration of exogenous estrogens for a prolonged time, long-duration surgical procedures, and bed rest in the postoperative period.[41]

A meta-analysis of studies on vaginoplasty outcomes that included 3,716 transgender women,[32] showed that the most frequent complications of vaginoplasty techniques include: stenosis (14%), fistula (1%), tissue necrosis (2%) and prolapse (4%). Another meta-analysis, with 1,684 cases, reports an overall complication rate of 32.5% with a reoperation rate of 21.7%, pointing to the same type of complications mentioned above.[33]

Overall satisfaction, assessed by the individuals themselves, was 92%, the degree of satisfaction related to function was 86%, and satisfaction with aesthetic appearance was 90%. The ability to have an orgasm was reported in 76% of cases. The dimensions of the vaginal cavity averaged 12.2 cm.[32]

The values of the scores obtained on quality of life scales increased after the surgery.

6.2.2. Breast reconstruction surgery

Breast reconstruction and augmentation surgery in transgender women is relatively similar to breast implant surgery performed in cisgender female individuals. The type, size and location of the implant depends on the increase of the mammary gland that was obtained with the gender-affirming hormone treatment. Sometimes fat grafts are used in conjunction with the implant to make it less visible and palpable and to decrease the cleavage plane between the two breasts. If the necessary increase is small, the fat graft may be sufficient.[36,34]

The American Society of Plastic Surgeons reported[35] that the complication rate for this surgery is relatively low, with the risk of serious complications or death being extremely low. Among the main complications are: hemorrhage, calcifications, fat embolism, fat necrosis, infection, cysts and loss of graft volume. Moreover, fat grafts do not appear to increase the risk of breast cancer or delay its detection by imaging means.

6.2.3. Facial feminization surgery

Usually the female face is more oval and with smoother lines compared to the male face, which has a more square structure and more angular lines. Facial feminization surgery performed by female transgender people may include chin reduction, modification of the jaw joint, reducing its angulation, reduction rhinoplasty, which may include lifting the tip of the nose, lip augmentation, forehead modification and frontal bossing, and capillary reimplantation, modifying the hairline.[36,37,38]

6.2.4. Chondrolaryngoplasty and voice surgery

The alteration of the tone of voice, making it higher pitched, can be obtained through several surgical techniques that shorten or increase the tension of the vocal cords. The Isshiki technique,[39] frequently used, fixes the thyroid and cricoid cartilages to each other through sutures, increasing the tension of the vocal cords. At the same time, a reduction of the thyroid cartilage can be performed. Surgical recovery is usually uncomplicated and the results are satisfactory. Transient voice weakness may occur due to prolonged edema.[36]

6.2.5. Orchiectomy

Orchiectomy can be performed in conjunction with vaginoplasty or before vaginal reconstruction surgery. It is very important that fertility preservation options have been discussed and implemented before performing this procedure.

6.3. Male gender affirmation surgeries

Male gender affirmation surgeries, as mentioned for female gender affirmation surgeries, aim on the one hand at the excision of the female sexual organs, hysterectomy, vaginectomy and salpingo-oophorectomy, and on the other hand, the reconstruction of male external sexual organs, phalloplasty, scrotoplasty and a masculinization of the body and face.

6.3.1. Facial masculinization surgery

Facial masculinization surgery is infrequent. Its objective is to reproduce facial and cranial features typical of the male sex, which include an increase in the transverse and longitudinal forehead, and the frontal prominence, chin and jaw projection, giving it a more square appearance, rhinoplasty and cheek augmentation.

In 2017, the first facial masculinization surgery was described together with a new procedure to create greater protuberance of the thyroid cartilage. The described procedure is based on the use of a costal cartilage graft in the thyroid cartilage.[40]

6.3.2. Chest masculinization

Bilateral mastectomy is the most frequently performed surgical procedure by male transgender people, and is often the only surgery these people want to undergo. There are several types of procedures taking into account breast size, nipple-areola implantation and breast ptosis. The choice of procedure should take into account not only breast removal but also reconstruction of the nipple area and removal of excess skin. The quality and appearance of the skin after surgery is one of the crucial aspects for the total success of the procedure.

6.3.3. Phalloplasty

Penis reconstruction, beyond the aesthetic aspect of the new organ, aims to preserve clitoral sensitivity, achieve erectile and tactile function allowing penetration during sexual intercourse, and enable the urinary function while standing. Another important aspect is minimizing consequences at the tissue donation site.[36,41,42]

There are several types of surgical approaches, with the use of a free forearm flap being the surgery that has gained the greatest consensus.[43] The forearm skin is thin and elastic, allowing a tube-within-a-tube configuration, creating a competent neourethra that enables bladder emptying while standing. The flap nerves are connected to the ilioinguinal nerve and dorsal nerve of the clitoris, providing tactile and erogenous sensitivity to the phallus. The clitoris is incorporated into the new penis in such a way that an orgasm is possible when stimulated.[36,44]

One of the main disadvantages of phalloplasty with a free forearm flap is the visible, sometimes stigmatizing scar on the forearm. A systematic review of the results of this surgical technique evaluated data from 665 individuals, with a mean follow-up of 6 years; 70% of individuals were satisfied with the aesthetic results, 69% reported having erogenous sensitivity, 77% tactile sensitivity, 75% were able to urinate while standing, and 42.5% reported having penetrative sexual intercourse.[45]

Alternatively, the surgery can be performed using a free or pedicled flap from the anterolateral thigh region, which has the advantage of being a less exposed area and therefore where a scar will be less visible. However, the skin is less thin and flexible, not allowing the same type of surgical plasticity regarding the redefinition of a neourethra. Other types of surgery use peroneal osteocutaneous flaps,[46] dorsal musculocutaneous flaps,[47] or abdominal tissue flaps.[48]

Urological complications of phalloplasty are relatively frequent, occurring in 40% to 50% of cases, and include fistulas and urethral stenosis.[49]

The implantation of testicular prostheses is an additional surgical procedure and is usually performed about a year after phalloplasty to allow complete healing of all tissues and enable the best conditions for the implant, with the lowest probability of complications. The scrotum can be reconstructed from flaps of the labia majora, whose skin texture and appearance are similar.[36]

6.3.4. Metoidioplasty

Metoidioplasty is a technique that consists of reconstructing a microphallus from a hypertrophied clitoris. The surgical procedure involves detaching the clitoris from the pubic bone and suspending and repositioning the urethra to accompany the microphallus.[50]

Sometimes metoidioplasty surgery is performed simultaneously with vaginectomy and hysterectomy, in a step preceding a subsequent phalloplasty surgery. The two-stage surgery minimizes the risk of blood loss, anemia, and possible loss of the flap used in phalloplasty.[36]

This surgery does not allow the person to have penetrative sexual intercourse or guarantee the ability to urinate while standing.

The aforementioned systematic review also analyzed the results of this surgical technique, including data from 378 individuals, with a mean follow-up of 4.6 years; 87% of individuals were satisfied with the aesthetic results, 100% reported having erogenous sensitivity, 89% were able to urinate while standing, and 0.5% reported having penetrative sexual intercourse.[45]

6.3.5. Vaginectomy

Vaginectomy can be performed simultaneously with phalloplasty or metoidioplasty. It is a delicate procedure, and its main complications are hemorrhage and the possibility of rectal perforation.[36]

6.3.6. Hysterectomy and Salpingo-oophorectomy

Hysterectomy can be performed abdominally or vaginally and/or laparoscopically. Sometimes a bilateral salpingo-oophorectomy is performed concomitantly with the hysterectomy. Performing these surgical techniques depends on the transgender person's wishes, but it may have the benefit of reducing the levels of testosterone administered, as there is a suppression of endogenous estrogen production. Another issue that has been considered is the risk of polycystic ovary syndrome, which could be increased in these individuals by long-term exposure to testosterone, but the available evidence is limited.

In people who do not undergo uterus and ovary removal, special attention should be given to monitoring for uterine, cervical, endometrial, and ovarian cancer.

Bibliography

[1] Grumbach M. M. The neuroendocrinology of human puberty revisited. Hormone research in paediatrics. 2002; 57(Suppl. 2): 2-14.

[2] Standards of Care for the Health of Transsexual, Transgender, and Gender NonconformingPeople. https://www.wpath.org/media/cms/Documents/Web%20Transfer/SOC/Sta ndards%20of%20Care%20V7%20-%202011%20WPATH.pdf [Accessed in 14/4/18].

[3] Unger C. A. Hormone therapy for transgender patients. Translational andrology and urology.

2016 Dec; 5(6): 877.

[4] Hembree W. C., Cohen-Kettenis P., Delemarre-Van De Waal H. A., Gooren L. J., Meyer IIIW. J., Spack N. P., Tangpricha V., Montori V. M. Endocrine treatment of transsexual persons: an Endocrine Society clinical

practice guideline. The Journal of Clinical Endocrinology & Metabolism. 2009 Sep 1; 94(9): 3132-54.

[5] Transgender women: Evaluation and management – UpToDate. https://www-uptodate-com. ezproxy.ub.unimaas.nl/contents/transgender-women-evaluation-and-management?search=transgender&source=search_result&selectedTitle=1~51&usage_type=default&display_rank=1#H10 [Accessed in 14/4/18].

[6] Asscheman H., T'Sjoen G., Lemaire A., et al. Venous thrombo-embolism as a complication of cross-sex hormone treatment of male-to-female transsexual subjects: a review. Andrologia. 2014; 46: 791.

[7] Center of Excellence for Transgender Health DoFaCM, UCSF. Guidelines for the Primary and Gender-Affirming Care of Transgender and Gender Nonbinary People: Center of

Excellence for Transgender Health, Department of Family and Community Medicine University of California San Francisco; 2016 2nd: www.transhealth.ucsf.edu/guidelines. [Accessed in 24/4/18].

[8] Connelly, P. J., Marie Freel, E., Perry, C., Ewan, J., Touyz, R. M., Currie, G., & Delles, C. (2019). Gender-Affirming Hormone Therapy, Vascular Health and Cardiovascular Disease in Transgender Adults. Hypertension (Dallas, Tex.: 1979), 74(6), 1266-1274. https://doi.org//10.1161/HYPERTENSIONAHA.119.13080.

[9] Radix A. (2019). Hormone Therapy for Transgender Adults. The Urologic clinics of North America, 46(4), 467-473. https://doi.org/10.1016/j.ucl.2019.07.001.

[10] Hembree W., Cohen-Kettenis P., Gooren L. Endocrine Treatment of Gender-Dysphoric/ /Gender-Incongruent Persons: An Endocrine Society Clinical Practice Guideline. J Clin Endocrinol Metab. 2017; 102(11): 3869-3903.

[11] de Bruin M. D., Coerts M. J., Greven A. J. Speech therapy in the management of male-tofemale transsexuals. Folia Phoniatr Logop. 2000; 52: 220.

[12] Hancock A. B., Garabedian L. M. Transgender voice and communication treatment: a retrospective chart review of 25 cases. Int J Lang Commun Disord. 2013; 48: 54.

[13] Asscheman H., Giltay E. J., Megens J. A., et al. A long-term follow-up study of mortality in transsexuals receiving treatment with cross-sex hormones. Eur J Endocrinol. 2011; 164: 635.

[14] Wierckx K., Elaut E., Declercq E., et al. Prevalence of cardiovascular disease and cancer during cross-sex hormone therapy in a large cohort of trans persons: a case-control study. Eur J Endocrinol. 2013; 169: 471.

[15] Goh H. H., Li X. F., Ratnam S. S. Effects of cross-gender steroid hormone treatment on prolactin concentrations in humans. Gynecol Endocrinol Off J Int Soc Gynecol Endocrinol.1992 Jun; 6(2): 113-7.

[16] Freda P. U., Beckers A. M., Katznelson L., Molitch M. E., Montori V. M., Post K. D., et al. Pituitary incidentaloma: an endocrine society clinical practice guideline. J Clin Endocrinol Metab. 2011 Apr; 96(4): 894-904.

[17] Gardner I. H., Safer J. D. Progress on the road to better medical care for transgender patients. Current Opinion in Endocrinology, Diabetes and Obesity. 2013 Dec 1; 20(6): 553-8.

[18] Practical Guidelines for Transgender Hormone Treatment https://www.bumc.bu.edu/endo//clinics/transgender-medicine/guidelines/ [Accessed in 14/4/18].

[19] Olson J., Forbes C., Belzer M. Management of the transgender adolescent. Archives of pediatrics & adolescent medicine. 2011 Feb 7; 165(2): 171-6.

[20] Transgender men: Evaluation and management – UpToDate. https://www-uptodate-com. ezproxy.ub.unimaas.nl/contents/transgender-men-evaluation-and-management?search=

transgender&source=search_result&selectedTitle=2~51&usage_type=default&display_rank=2#H4223768816 [Accessed in 14/4/18].

[21] Irwig M. S. Testosterone therapy for transgender men. The Lancet Diabetes & Endocrinology. 2017 Apr 1; 5(4): 301-11.

[22] Wierckx K., Mueller S., Weyers S., Van Caenegem E., Roef G., Heylens G., T'sjoen G. Long-term evaluation of cross-sex hormone treatment in transsexual persons. The journal of sexual medicine. 2012 Oct 1; 9(10): 2641-51.

[23] Weinand J. D., Safer J. D. Hormone therapy in transgender adults is safe with provider supervision; A review of hormone therapy sequelae for transgender individuals. J Clin Transl Endocrinol. 2015; 2: 55.

[24] Gardner I. H., Safer J. D. Progress on the road to better medical care for transgender patients. Current Opinion in Endocrinology, Diabetes and Obesity. 2013 Dec 1; 20(6): 553-8.

[25] Practical Guidelines for Transgender Hormone Treatment https://www.bumc.bu.edu/endo//clinics/transgender-medicine/guidelines/ [Accessed in 14/4/18].

[26] Olson J., Forbes C., Belzer M. Management of the transgender adolescent. Archives of pediatrics & adolescent medicine. 2011 Feb 7; 165(2): 171-6.

[27] Colizzi M., Costa R., Pace V., Todarello O. Hormonal treatment reduces psychobiological distress in gender identity disorder, independently of the attachment style. The journal of sexual medicine. 2013 Dec 1; 10(12): 3049-58.

[28] Kranz G. S., Wadsak W., Kaufmann U., Savli M., Baldinger P., Gryglewski G., Haeusler D., Spies M., Mitterhauser M., Kasper S., Lanzenberger R. High-dose testosterone treatment increases serotonin transporter binding in transgender people. Biological psychiatry. 2015 Oct 15; 78(8): 525-33.

[29] Karim R. B., Hage J. J., Bouman F. G., et al. Refinements of pre-, intra-, and postoperative care to prevent complications of vaginoplasty in male transsexuals. Ann Plast Surg. 1995; 35: 279-284.

[30] Manrique O. J., Sabbagh M. D., Ciudad P., et al. Gender confirmation surgery using the pedicle transverse colon flap for vaginal reconstruction: a clinical outcome and sexual function evaluation study. Plast Reconstr Surg. 2017; 11

[31] Transgender surgery: Male to female – UpToDate https://www-uptodate-com.ezproxy.ub. unimaas.nl/contents/transgender-surgery-male-to-female?search=transgender&source=search_result&selectedTitle=5~51&usage_type=default&display_rank=5 [Accessed in 14/4/18].

[32] Manrique O. J., Adabi K., Martinez-Jorge J., Nicoli F., Kiranantawat K. Complications and Patient-Reported Outcomes in Male-to-Female Vaginoplasty-Where We Are Today: A Systematic Review and Meta-Analysis. Annals of plastic surgery. 2018 Feb.

[33] Dreher P. C., Edwards D., Hager S., Dennis M., Belkoff A., Mora J., Tarry S., Rumer K. L. Complications of the Neovagina in Male-to-Female Transgender Surgery: A Systematic Review and Meta-analysis with Discussion of Management. Clinical Anatomy. 2017 Oct 23.

[34] Wesp L. M., Deutsch M. B. Hormonal and surgical treatment options for transgender women and transfeminine spectrum persons. Psychiatric Clinics. 2017 Mar 1; 40(1): 99-111.

[35] American Society of Plastic Surgeons. Post-mastectomy fat graft/fat transfer ASPS guiding principles. https://www.plasticsurgery.org/Documents/Health-Policy/Principles/principle-2015-post-mastectomy-fat-grafting.pdf [Accessed in 8/4/18].

[36] Colebunders B., Brondeel S., D'Arpa S., Hoebeke P., Monstrey S. An update on the surgical treatment for transgender patients. Sexual medicine reviews. 2017 Jan 1; 5(1): 103-9.

[37] Spiegel J. H. Challenges in care of the transgender patient seeking facial feminization surgery. Facial Plastic Surgery Clinics. 2008 May 1; 16(2): 233-8.

[38] Altman K. Facial feminization surgery: current state of the art. International journal of oral and maxillofacial surgery. 2012 Aug 1; 41(8): 885-94.

[39] Isshiki N., Taira T., Kojima H., et al. Recent modifications in thyroplasty type I. Ann Otol Rhinol Laryngol. 1989; 98: 777-779.

[40] Deschamps-Braly J. C., Sacher C. L., Fick J., Ousterhout D. K. First female-to-male facial confirmation surgery with description of a new procedure for masculinization of the thyroid cartilage (Adam's apple). Plastic and reconstructive surgery. 2017 Apr 1; 139(4): 883e-7e.

[41] Selvaggi G., Bellringer J. Gender reassignment surgery: an overview. Nature Reviews Urology. 2011 May; 8(5): 274.

[42] Morrison S. D., Perez M. G., Nedelman M., Crane C. N. Current state of female-to-male gender confirming surgery. Current Sexual Health Reports. 2015 Mar 1; 7(1): 38-48.

[43] Kim S., Dennis M., Holland J., Terrell M., Loukas M., Schober J. The anatomy of forearm free flap phalloplasty for transgender surgery. Clinical Anatomy. 2018 Mar 1; 31(2): 145-51.

[44] Morrison S. D., Perez M. G., Carter C. K., Crane C. N. Pre-and postoperative care with associated intra-operative techniques for phalloplasty in female-to-male patients. Urologic nursing. 2015 May 1; 35(3): 134-43.

[45] Frey J. D., Poudrier G., Chiodo M. V., Hazen A. A systematic review of metoidioplasty and radial forearm flap phalloplasty in female-to-male transgender genital reconstruction:

is the «ideal» neophallus an achievable goal? Plastic and Reconstructive Surgery Global Open. 2016 Dec; 4(12).

[46] Zaheer U., Granger A., Ortiz A., Terrell M., Loukas M., Schober J. The anatomy of free fibula osteoseptocutaneous flap in neophalloplasty in transgender surgery. Clinical Anatomy. 2018 Mar 1; 31(2): 169-74.

[47] Dennis M., Granger A., Ortiz A., Terrell M., Loukos M., Schober J. The anatomy of the musculocutaneous latissimus dorsi flap for neophalloplasty. Clinical Anatomy. 2018 Mar 1;

31(2): 152-9.

[48] Kim S., Dennis M., Holland J., Terrell M., Loukas M., Schober J. The anatomy of abdominal flap phalloplasty for transgender surgery. Clinical Anatomy. 2018 Mar 1; 31(2): 181-6.

[49] Santucci R. A. Urethral Complications after Transgender Phalloplasty and Strategies to Treat Them and Minimize Their Occurrence. Clinical Anatomy. 2017 Nov 27.

[50] Frey J. D., Poudrier G., Chiodo M. V., Hazen A. An update on genital reconstruction options

for the female-to-male transgender patient: a review of the literature. Plastic and reconstructive surgery. 2017 Mar 1; 139(3): 728-37.

Chapter 7 - Fertility Preservation in Transgender Individuals

Hormonal and surgical gender affirmation treatments have negative effects on fertility potential. Thus, it is essential to inform and discuss with each individual the consequences of the treatments and the options regarding future fertility. Although there are few studies on this topic, it is estimated that about half of transgender men[1] and half of transgender women[2] would like to have children. This fact is even more important considering that parenthood has a positive effect on the mental health and vitality of transgender people, having been considered as a protective factor against the risk of suicide in transgender women.[3]

According to the World Professional Association for Transgender Health (WPATH), fertility options should be discussed before any medical or surgical intervention.

The gender affirmation hormone therapy used in transgender women involves the prolonged use of estrogens. This results in a reduction in testicular volume, reduction in sperm motility and density. Although this effect may be reversible after treatment interruption, reversibility depends on the presence of viable spermatogonial stem cells.

Orchiectomy, a surgical option used in transgender women, leads to irreversible sterility.

Hormone therapy with testosterone in transgender men and increased androgens has a negative effect on ovarian follicular tissue. However, despite this negative effect, pregnancy is possible in individuals undergoing gender affirmation treatment with testosterone,[4,5] with the latter having teratogenic effects.

Transgender men undergoing hormone therapy with testosterone should consider using effective contraceptive methods, with the choice falling on the use of intrauterine devices or barrier methods.

Hysterectomy and bilateral oophorectomy lead to irreversible sterility.

Currently, options for fertility preservation in transgender men include cryopreservation of embryos, oocytes, or ovarian tissue.[6,7] In the first two cases, an ovarian stimulation treatment is performed, and oocytes are collected. This technique must be performed before testosterone hormone treatment (or after interrupting it for at least 3 months). The technique involves monitoring ovarian stimulation through transvaginal ultrasound and oocyte aspiration by transvaginal surgical procedure. The need for gynecological exams and transvaginal procedures can constitute an important factor of discomfort, anxiety, and stress, limiting the use of this procedure.

In the case of oocyte cryopreservation, after collection, the oocytes are cryopreserved without being fertilized, and in the future, they can be fertilized with donor sperm (or from a male partner), and this embryo can be implanted in the uterus of surrogate carriers or in the uterus of a female partner.

In the case of embryo cryopreservation, the process is similar to that described previously regarding oocyte cryopreservation, but fertilization is performed before the cryopreservation process.

Ovarian tissue cryopreservation is still an experimental technique and consists of the collection and cryopreservation of ovarian tissue, surgically harvested. In this technique, there is no need for ovarian stimulation. If applicable, ovarian tissue resection can be performed during oophorectomy, since undergoing hormone treatment with testosterone does not directly affect the potential of the ovarian tissue.

Currently, fertility preservation options for transgender women include sperm cryopreservation and immature testicular tissue cryopreservation.[6,7]

Sperm cryopreservation can be performed from a semen sample obtained by ejaculation (by masturbation) or through surgical sperm extraction, by percutaneous aspiration of sperm from the testicle or epididymis.

In either case, the sample is cryopreserved and can be used later for an in vitro fertilization process, with eggs from the partner if she is female or with donor eggs and the use of a surrogate carrier.

Immature testicular tissue cryopreservation is an experimental procedure in which a surgical biopsy of testicular tissue is performed. The surgical procedure can be performed concomitantly with gender affirmation surgery.

Bibliography

[1] Wierckx K., Van Caenegem E., Pennings G., Elaut E., Dedecker D., Van de Peer F., Weyers S., De Sutter P., T'sjoen G. Reproductive wish in transsexual men. Human Reproduction. 2011 Nov 28; 27(2): 483-7.

[2] Wierckx K., Stuyver I., Weyers S., Hamada A., Agarwal A., De Sutter P., T'Sjoen G. Sperm freezing in transsexual women. Archives of sexual behavior. 2012 Oct 1; 41(5): 1069-71.

[3] Hamada A., Kingsberg S., Wierckx K., T'Sjoen G., De Sutter P., Knudson G., Agarwal A. Semen characteristics of transwomen referred for sperm banking before sex transition: a case series. Andrologia. 2015 Sep 1; 47(7): 832-8.

[4] Light A. D., Obedin-Maliver J., Sevelius J. M., Kerns J. L. Transgender men who experienced pregnancy after female-to-male gender transitioning. Obstetrics & Gynecology. 2014 Dec 1; 124(6): 1120-7.

[5] T'Sjoen G., Van Caenegem E., Wierckx K. Transgenderism and reproduction. Current Opinion in Endocrinology, Diabetes and Obesity. 2013 Dec 1; 20(6): 575-9.

[6] Wallace S. A., Blough K. L., Kondapalli L. A. Fertility preservation in the transgender patient: expanding oncofertility care beyond cancer. Gynecological Endocrinology. 2014 Dec 1; 30(12): 868-71.

[7] De Roo C., Tilleman K., T'Sjoen G., De Sutter P. Fertility options in transgender people. International Review of Psychiatry. 2016 Jan 2; 28(1): 112-9.

Chapter 8 - Transgender Athletes: Competitive Sports and Doping

Most sports have a binary segmentation, with women's and men's events. This fact, in addition to being based on sociocultural reasons where male predominance and discrimination are still prevalent, is based on physical and physiological issues that determine differences between women and men.

Men have a muscle mass about 30% higher than that of women, which gives them more strength, power, and height. Women have more elastic muscle fibers. Thus, as physical characteristics favor results in certain types of sports, it is considered fairer for competitions to be divided based on sex.

Transgender people undergoing hormone replacement therapy pose a challenge to the sex dichotomy prevalent in sports. For years, transgender people were prevented from participating in competitive sports in which competition was divided into female and male categories, particularly in the Olympic Games. Over the past few years, there has been a modification of rules and regulations in order not to discriminate against transgender people and to find a way to promote their inclusion in fair competition.

In 2015, the International Olympic Committee rectified its position on this issue, after having issued very restrictive recommendations in 2003. In the 2015 recommendations, there is no impediment resulting from a person having undergone any type of gender affirmation surgery. It is expressed that individuals who transition or have transitioned from female to male are eligible to compete in male categories without restrictions. This criterion, although inclusive, is somewhat sexist since it is based on the assumption that a transgender man is at a disadvantage compared to cisgender men.

After the 2020 Olympic Games were the first with openly transgender athletes, in 2021 the Olympic Committee published a document entitled "IOC Framework on Fairness, Inclusion and Non-Discrimination on the Basis of Gender Identity and Sex Variations", changing the rules defined until then and based on respect for freedom and people, inclusion, and non-discrimination.

Until 2015, the Olympic Committee imposed that, for transgender women, testosterone levels were evaluated and had to have a value below 10 nmol/L for at least 12 months prior to the first competition and remained at these values during the competition period in female categories. In the new document, it is considered that testosterone levels are not the best way to assess the possibility of athletes competing in female categories, especially since different modalities and federations have different criteria.[1]

Another important aspect in the sports practice of transgender athletes concerns doping control and the need to obtain a Therapeutic Use Exemption (TUE) for the gender affirmation hormone therapies that are used. Testosterone used in transgender men and spironolactone used in transgender women are included in the list of substances prohibited by the World Anti-Doping Agency. Estrogens are not part of the list of prohibited substances. Gonadotropin-releasing hormone (GnRH) analogues are used in long-term treatments for transgender women. These substances are currently prohibited for male athletes since they have an initial effect of stimulating testosterone. Transgender female athletes eligible for participation in female events do not require a TUE for GnHR analogues. On the other hand, transgender female athletes in the process of feminization but who still compete in male events need to obtain a TUE for GnHR analogues.[2]

Since, in transgender men undergoing gender affirmation hormone therapy, testosterone is a treatment commonly used for life, the validity attributed to the TUE is 10 years, and it is mandatory to have annual follow-up reports that include the dose and regimen of testosterone administration and serum levels. Similarly, the validity of the TUE for spironolactone in transgender female individuals is also 10 years and requires annual follow-up reports.

Bibliography

[1]   https://olympics.com/ioc/news/ioc-releases-framework-on-fairness-inclusion-and-non--discrimination-on-the-basis-of-gender-identity-and-sex-variations [Accessed in 17-11-22].

[2] TUE PHYSICIAN GUIDELINES Medical Information to Support the Decisions of TUE Committees TRANSGENDER ATHLETES. https://www.wada-ama.org/sites/default/files/ /resources/files/wada_transgender_athletes_v1.0_en.pdf [Accessed in 14/4/18].

Chapter 9 - Health Specificities in the Lesbian, Gay and Bisexual Population

When addressing the topic of health specificities in the lesbian, gay and bisexual (LGB) population, there is a tendency to assume that, because LGB people have a different sexual orientation than the majority of individuals, they have specific diseases or more diseases than the general population. In most situations, this is not true. Sexual orientation per se does not translate into any specific pathological situation. However, there are situations in this group of people that should be approached in a specific way, either because they are more prevalent or because they are associated with other potentially modifiable external factors.

The main cause of health disparities in the LGB population is lower access to and inadequate provision of health care. For decades, and still today, the LGB population has suffered some degree of discrimination by health services and professionals. This discrimination can be explicit, sometimes even homophobic, or it can simply be discrimination based on ignorance and the inability to communicate in a way that obtains the crucial elements for a complete clinical assessment. If the medical team treating the ill person does not always consider the possibility that they may not be heterosexual, the probability of the approach being heteronormative is extremely high.

When confronting a lesbian woman with questions or statements like "your husband..." or a gay man with "your wife...", an environment of discomfort, distrust and non-inclusion is immediately created, which in most situations is decisive for the person not to expose themselves. This "closing" movement by LGB patients causes the omission of many facts and can lead to inappropriate clinical practice. On the other hand, by feeling uncomfortable, LGB people tend to avoid and postpone seeking medical care. This increases, for example, the likelihood of not having screenings and thus increases the prevalence of neoplastic disease in this segment of the population.

Having at every moment and with every patient the awareness that sexual orientation is an issue that should not be assumed from the outset and that it is a question that must be asked and whose answer is useful in clinical thinking, is a fundamental step for equity in health care in the LGB population.

Equity of health care in the LGB population does not mean equal health care to that of the heterosexual population, it means equal health care in everything that is similar and differentiated and appropriate care in everything that is specific to this group of people.

LGB people often face, throughout their lives, a greater or lesser degree of discrimination. This discrimination, or the potential for it to happen even if it is not present, is in itself a strong anxiety factor. Thus, anxiety disorders, mood disorders or addictive behaviors should be considered.

Finally, a reference to sexually transmitted diseases. When talking about LGB health, one of the issues that arises almost immediately is HIV infection. Many medical school curricula only address the topic of sexual orientation in the nosological context of AIDS. Sexually transmitted diseases depend on the type of sexual behavior of the individual. This does not mean that they depend on their sexual orientation. For example, a homosexual man with a single stable partner (who also has a single partner) is not at greater risk for sexually transmitted diseases than a heterosexual man with a single partner and will certainly have less risk than a heterosexual man with multiple partners.

However, it is important not to neglect that sexual behavior, especially of homosexual men, is often a risky behavior due on one hand to the fact that they have multiple partners and on the other hand to the fact that they do not use protection methods during sex. Again, it should be taken into account that the risk is not associated with the person being homosexual but rather with them having multiple partners or other risk behaviors.

A group to consider in the assessment of risk for sexually transmitted diseases is that of men who have sex with men (MSM), without identifying as homosexual and, in some situations, without even identifying as bisexual. These individuals usually have several partners, with whom they have little intimacy, and the sexual relationship is fortuitous. In this context, the risk of sexually transmitted diseases is increased.

9.1. Intersectionality

Intersectionality is a conceptual matrix based on the concept that individuals have multiple identities that overlap and that only the analysis of these identities and their relationships allows avoiding inequity, namely with regard to health. In social terms, the concept suggests that practices such as racism, sexism, classism, homophobia or transphobia do not act independently of each other, interrelating and creating a system of discrimination.[1] Moreover, when these people interact with the educational, legal or health system, they tend to be and feel marginalized, which constitutes another form of discrimination.

Although the concept of intersectionality has been developed in a social context, it has direct applicability in health. If we consider that some pathological situations have a higher prevalence in individuals with a certain sexual orientation or gender identity, we must question whether it is a direct causal relationship or whether we are facing an intersectionality network.

For example, if being male implies a higher probability of being a smoker, if being a homosexual person implies a higher probability of being a smoker, and if having a lower level of education also implies a higher probability of being a smoker, then a homosexual male individual with a low level of education will have a higher risk of lung cancer. Lung cancer has tobacco as a causal factor and not sexual orientation or gender, but it is still associated with these variables. In terms of health care, this can be decisive, because if we are aware of the multiple relationships and variables that are directly or indirectly related to a given pathology, we can act preventively.

The following subchapters address several pathologies and risk factors that have been described as having their own specificities in the LGB group. It should be noted that for many of the topics the available evidence is limited. Despite this, and in case of uncertainty, it is always preferable to consider the possibility of increased risk or any specificity in relation to a given pathology, keeping this in mind during the collection of clinical history, physical examination, complementary tests and diagnostic guidance.

9.2. Clinical history and physical examination in lesbian, gay or bisexual people

The clinical approach to LGB people is similar to that of any person. However, it is important to pay special attention not to hurt susceptibilities or create situations of discomfort and breakdown of trust, which can result from the use of a heteronormative discourse. The use of open-ended questions, without value judgments or established standards, is important for a fluid and true conversation.

One should not assume a person's sexual orientation based on their physical appearance and behavior. Appearance mainly reflects the gender expression with which the person identifies and not their sexual orientation. For any person, it should be assumed that they may be heterosexual, homosexual, bisexual, pansexual or asexual and, whatever their identification, the possibility of sexual relations, fortuitous or not, with any persons regardless of their sex and gender should not be excluded. For example, it is relatively common for heterosexual men to have had sexual relations with men. This fact is important to the extent that it can increase the risk of certain pathologies and this should be taken into account in the management of the clinical situation.

From the above, it follows that sexual orientation should be asked about and not assumed by the medical team. If the person being evaluated has a sexual orientation that is assumed for themselves and for others, the collection of this aspect of the clinical history will be easier and more direct. But many people have not (yet) assumed their sexual orientation to third parties or to society in general, so they may tend to lie or omit information during a clinical evaluation. The fear of being discriminated against overrides the risk of a less correct health assessment, due to lack of information or inadequate information.

The collection of sexual history should be done gradually, openly and in a gender neutral way. The history should be adapted according to the person being evaluated, especially if they are young adolescents.

Clinical approach and history taking are often performed in the presence of third parties, that is, the ill person comes to the consultation or the emergency room accompanied by their mother, partner, child or sister, who attend the consultation and sometimes even participate by giving information and even transmitting their own opinion. This can be good, but it can lead the ill person not to express themselves. Before addressing any questions about sexual orientation, it is important to try to understand the degree of intimacy and information sharing between the ill person and the accompanying person. The ill person should be explicitly asked, whenever they are of legal age and even in adolescents, depending on the context, if they feel more comfortable conducting the consultation alone. If they express this desire, the accompanying person should be asked to wait a little outside the room, but if the ill person says they prefer the presence of the other, their preference should be respected.

Sexual history also includes inquiring about symptoms or signs of sexually transmitted diseases, explicitly and even giving examples to ensure that the question is well understood. For example, one should ask directly if the person has vaginal, penile or anal discharge, dysuria, dyspareunia, genital lesions or pain during sex. It should also be assessed whether the person has ever had a diagnosis of STD.

Gynecological history should be collected, including menstrual history, contraception and pregnancy.

In the case of gay or lesbian individuals or couples, fertility and parenting issues should be addressed specifically and are focused on in a later chapter - Parenting and pregnancy in homosexual couples or individuals.

The physical examination of LGB individuals is no different from other physical exams, with the exception of the gynecological examination of lesbian women. For a lesbian woman, especially if she has never had vaginal penetrative intercourse, the gynecological exam, both the insertion of the speculum and the bimanual exam, can be very uncomfortable and painful.

Before starting the gynecological exam, the procedure that will be performed should be described and it should be noted that it can be interrupted whenever necessary. It is important to try to obtain maximum relaxation, as this will facilitate the examination. In the speculum exam, a pediatric speculum can be used that allows visualization of the cervix and vaginal walls with less discomfort for the woman.

The fear on the part of lesbian individuals regarding gynecological exams often leads to avoidance of these visits and, consequently, failure to perform cervical cancer screening and even breast cancer screening.

9.3. Coming out - Addressing sexual orientation with parents of lesbian, gay or bisexual youth

The age at which each person becomes aware of their sexual orientation is extremely variable and, throughout life, one's opinion on the subject may not be constant.

When an adolescent becomes aware that they are homosexual or bisexual, there is a first phase of internalizing the situation and reflecting on it, sometimes done individually, other times done with friends or with a first boyfriend/girlfriend. This phase can cause feelings of anxiety, anguish or fear, discomfort with one's own sexuality and with others, or even an internal feeling of homophobia.

Sharing information about sexuality with parents (The text refers to "parents" since it is the most frequent family model for most adolescents.

However, throughout the text, parents should be understood as caregivers, and may be a single mother or father, grandparents, uncles or other adults responsible for the adolescent, with whom they share daily life.) is usually uncomfortable for any adolescent, regardless of their sexual orientation. For LGB youth, the situation is even more difficult, because in addition to addressing a somewhat embarrassing topic, by sharing a homosexual, bisexual, pansexual or asexual sexual orientation, they anticipate a potentially less positive reaction.

Sharing with family and their acceptance are extremely important vectors for the health of the young person. Rejection reactions from the family have been shown to be directly related to the risk of suicide, with an 8-fold increased risk, the risk of depression and the risk of drug abuse, with a 6-fold and 3-fold increased risk, respectively.[2]

An analysis conducted in the United States in 2012[3] evaluated 10,000 youth between the ages of 13 and 17 who identified as LGBT and showed that 56% of youth had shared their sexual orientation with their parents/family.

The sharing of sexual orientation with parents or other family members must be done by the person themselves. However, the medical team may be confronted either by the individual who asks for help in the best way to "have this conversation", or by the parents, who often anticipate the situation, due to behaviors or attitudes of the young person, but have never talked about the subject.

The most important attitude is to convey that sexual orientation is not in itself a clinical issue. It is not a pathology and should never be seen as such. An adolescent being homosexual is as normal and "natural" as being heterosexual or bisexual, being different ways of feeling and expressing sexuality.

Both parents and adolescents should be aware that sharing information and living it transparently, with support and normalcy, in the family and social context, is extremely beneficial for the healthy growth and development of the adolescent. Part of this experience is the deconstruction of heteronormative patterns and, often, for parents, the learning of a new language and form of communication that is inclusive and non-discriminatory.

In some situations, parents react negatively, not because they are homophobic people, but because they anticipate that their children may suffer social discrimination that affects their future life. The internalized fear that their children will suffer, together with the anxiety caused by anticipating what their children's sexual orientation may condition in their own lives, are enough to trigger aggressive responses to the situation. It is important to promote parents' awareness in these circumstances of the fact that they themselves are being aggressors, when they should be the main support.

In clinical terms, there are situations that are more frequent in LGB people as a group. Individually, younger people should be alerted to possible risk behaviors, which are no different from those for which any young person (and adult) should be alerted, regardless of their sexual orientation.

9.4. Parenting and pregnancy in homosexual couples or individuals

Couples of homosexual individuals, or homosexual individuals themselves, often, and increasingly, express the desire to be mothers/fathers. In these cases, the medical team should be able to provide information about available alternatives.

Homosexual individuals can become mothers or fathers through adoption, medically assisted procreation (MAP) techniques, in the case of women, and surrogacy.

In the case of MAP, the lesbian couple, or the lesbian woman, should be referred to a reference center, which will follow the process from the beginning. The techniques used in MAP include intrauterine insemination (IUI) and in vitro fertilization (IVF). The MAP process itself does not differ because it is a homoparental family, beyond the use of donor sperm.2

Although evidence regarding the results of MAP techniques specifically in lesbian individuals is limited, studies that have addressed this issue have shown overlapping results when comparing pregnancy rates in lesbian and heterosexual women of similar ages and without criteria for infertility or subfertility.

Several studies show that since most women who resort to MAP techniques do so due to infertility or subfertility situations, their results tend to be worse than those obtained by lesbian women, usually without previous pathology. Other factors that may determine a difference in outcomes between lesbian and heterosexual women include personal and social context and the prevalence of some risk factors such as obesity or smoking, in addition to the woman's age at the time she seeks pregnancy.

The results of the studies show distinct conclusions that mainly reflect the baseline characteristics of the women included. In a study published in 2008,[8] De Sutter reported statistically similar results in the pregnancy rate obtained in women from lesbian and heterosexual couples, 60% versus 55%, respectively, after an average of 3 IUI cycles. In 2014,[9] a study conducted in Sweden analyzed MAP results in 171 lesbian women and 124 heterosexual women. The percentage of women who had babies was similar in both groups, being 69% and 72%, respectively, in lesbian and heterosexual women. The average number of treatments performed was also similar, being 3.9 for lesbian women and 4.2 for heterosexual women. The percentage of pregnancy per IUI cycle was 20.5% for lesbian women and 18.4% for heterosexual women. The percentage of pregnancy per IVF cycle was 32% for both groups, with slightly higher values when analyzing IVF performed with fresh embryos.

A meta-analysis, published in 2017,[10] analyzed pregnancy in lesbian women and heterosexual women and concluded that, overall, pregnancy is much less frequent in lesbian women than in heterosexual women, with an OR of 0.12 (which represents about nine times less). On the other hand, the same study describes a higher success rate in MAP situations for lesbian women, with an OR of 1.56.

It is important to keep in mind that the surrounding conditions, the context, are important. In most health care settings where prenatal and postnatal care is provided, including maternity hospitals, the environment tends to be very heteronormative. That is, almost everything is predetermined according to the existence of a mother and a father, from the language used by health professionals to forms, posters decorating the walls, or informative leaflets. The creation of inclusive and non-discriminatory environments is important for the well-being of all those involved, contributing to the optimization of the health care provided.

9.5. Approach to same-sex parent families

Same-sex parent families are made up of one or more children of two lesbian mothers or two gay fathers. This designation also includes single-parent families consisting of a lesbian mother and one or more children, or a gay father and one or more children, and situations of homosexual couples in which one of the members of the couple has children from a previous relationship.

During the last decades, several studies have been carried out, including meta-analyses, that evaluated the cognitive and emotional development of children of homosexual couples, with the overall conclusion that there are no differences in development compared to children of heterosexual parents.

A meta-analysis published in 2007[11] included 19 studies and compared the results of children of homosexual and heterosexual mothers/fathers regarding child development and well-being and the relationship between mothers (or fathers) and the child. No differences were found regarding the child's cognitive development, gender expression, gender identity, psychological adjustment or sexual orientation. Regarding the relationship between mothers/fathers and child, it had significantly better results for homosexual couples compared to heterosexual couples.

A study published in 2016[12] analyzed data from the 2013 National Health Interview Survey in the United States, comparing matched results from 95 same-sex parent and different-sex parent families with children between 6 and 17 years old. The study concluded there were no differences in any of the evaluated parameters, in health in general, emotional difficulties, coping strategies, learning, family relationship, with the exception of stress levels of mothers/fathers, which were higher in same-sex parent families.

The clinical approach to same-sex parent families should seek to be inclusive and not heteronormative. The language used should be appropriate, referring to mothers or fathers in the plural and not trying to identify if one or the other member of the couple is "more" mother or father than the other. Sometimes in lesbian couples who had a child through the pregnancy of one of the members of the couple, by ART techniques, there may be a tendency to consider that the mother, "in the true sense of the term", is the person who was pregnant. This attitude is disruptive for the couple and can be strange for the child from a certain age.

In terms of a more global approach, inclusion should be promoted in all environments that the child attends, encouraging the use of appropriate language. One should try to find out how the child identifies each of their two mothers or two fathers and respect the nomenclature chosen by the child and used by the family.

The informed, inclusive and non-discriminatory participation of the school is essential for the child to have an adequate development. In this context, it is important to share with the other children and educators that families of two mothers or two fathers are the same as families with a mother and a father, only a mother or only a father, or with grandparents or uncles. In reality, it is essential to promote knowledge of proximity and even some degree of intimacy so that all families are seen as equal and equally normal.

The inclusion of same-sex parent families in children's books, animated series or movies is essential so that all children with this type of family identify with their favorite characters and, on the other hand, so that all children can have contact with this reality and, increasingly, diversity becomes part of our normality.

9.6. Smoking

In general, studies point to higher tobacco consumption starting at younger ages in the LGB population compared to the general population. However, it is not likely that sexual orientation itself increases the risk of smoking, but rather other factors that are associated with sexual orientation on the one hand and with smoking on the other.

Whether or not the association between sexual orientation and smoking is direct, it is important to consider that, since tobacco is one of the risk factors most associated with cardiovascular disease and cancer, any smoker is at greater risk for these pathologies and their clinical approach should take this into consideration.

In European countries the evidence available regarding the prevalence of smoking taking sexual orientation into account is relatively limited.

A study published in 2013[13] in the Irish population, which included 635 people who identified as LGB, points to a higher prevalence of smokers in LGB people than in the general population in Ireland, 45% versus 29%. The estimated weighted prevalence value for lesbian people was 46%, being 45% for gay men and 45% for people who identified as bisexual.

Another study from 2014[14] regarding the Swedish population evaluated 24,348 people and found a smoking prevalence of 13.5% (14.8% in women and 11.9% in men) in the general population. Approximately 3%, 730 of the evaluated individuals, identified as LGB. In these, the prevalence of smoking was 11.3% in lesbian women, 23.6% in bisexual women, 22.4% in gay men and 22.2% in bisexual men.

A study conducted in the United States, published in 2018[15], evaluated 265 lesbian women, 422 bisexual women, 19,454 heterosexual women and 321 gay men, 144 bisexual men and 15,190 heterosexual men, and found a smoking prevalence of 21% in heterosexual women, 37% in lesbian women and 46% in bisexual women. In men, the prevalence found was 33% for heterosexual men, 37% for gay men and 50% for bisexual men. Although, in general, the prevalence of smoking is higher in both men and women who identify as homosexual versus those who identify as heterosexual, this is not the case in the age group 55 years or older. In people who identify as bisexual, the prevalence is higher in all age groups.

A review published in 2011[16], which sought to analyze factors that correlated with smoking in LGB people, found a large disparity between the results of the analyzed studies (the analyzed studies were conducted in the United States, Australia and Mexico). The main factors associated with an increased prevalence of smoking were those that are also associated with smoking in heterosexual individuals and include: younger age, lower education, alcohol consumption and presence of depressive symptoms or depression.[17,18] Victimization or presence of discriminatory factors did not show a conclusive association with smoking,[19,20] but are risk factors associated with increased risk of mental illness. Other factors analyzed included self-concept and negative attitudes of the self towards homosexuality or rejection by the family.[21] These factors also showed mixed results between studies, and their association with smoking was not conclusive.

A meta-analysis published in 2020, which included 147 studies, compared the lifetime prevalence of smoking in people with different sexual orientations, concluding that, compared to lesbian or gay people and heterosexual people, bisexual people are 1.25 (95% CI 1.15 to 1.37) and 2.18 (95% CI 1.84 to 2.59) times more likely to be smokers.[22]

9.7. Alcohol and drug use

Historically, alcohol and drug use has been described as having a higher frequency in LGB people, but some reviews on this topic show that the results are mixed and depend on the type of populations evaluated and especially that they are associated with the surrounding personal and sociocultural context. Age, gender, bisexuality, stress level and HIV infection have been shown to be associated with patterns of alcohol and drug use in LGB people. Older age and female gender act as protective factors, that is, of lower risk, in heterosexual people. However, this does not seem to be the case in homosexual people. In heterosexual people, male individuals usually have higher and more frequent consumption compared to female individuals. This difference seems to be much less pronounced in LGB people.[23] In this group of people, bisexual people tend to be those with the highest frequency of alcohol consumption.

A study conducted in Sweden, published in 2017[24], analyzed alcohol and cannabis use in people registered in the Swedish National Public Health Survey, between 2008 and 2015, aged between 16 and 84 years, according to sexual orientation. The results showed a prevalence of alcohol consumption, designated as high risk5, in 16.4% of heterosexual people, 25.2% of homosexual people and 20.3% of bisexual people. Regarding cannabis use in the previous 12 months, the frequencies were 1.4%, 4.3% and 7.7%, respectively. This study also showed that there is a strong association between alcohol and cannabis use and levels of psychological stress, especially in LGB people.

An analysis carried out in the United States population over 18 years of age, based on data from the 2013-14 National Health Interview Survey[25], showed that the prevalence of high-risk alcohol consumption6 was higher in LGB people compared to heterosexual people with the same characteristics. The frequencies of people with high-risk alcohol consumption were 5.7% for heterosexual men, 5.1% for gay men and 10.9% for bisexual men.

For women, the frequencies were 4.8% for heterosexual women, 8.9% for lesbian women, and 11.7% for bisexual women. In relative terms, the OR values were 1.97 for gay men and 3.15 for bisexual men versus heterosexual men, and 2.63 and 2.07, respectively, for lesbian women and bisexual women versus heterosexual women.

A study published in 2018[26] analyzed alcohol and drug use in the adolescent population of the United States, comparing the results according to the sexual orientation of the youth. The prevalence of alcohol consumption and marijuana use were similar in gay and bisexual youth compared to heterosexual youth. The only difference found in this study was in the use of prescription drugs, which was significantly higher in gay youth (RR 1.97) compared to heterosexual youth. In young women, the use of prescription drugs was higher in lesbian youth compared to heterosexual youth (RR 1.58). Bisexual young women reported higher consumption of alcohol, illicit drugs and prescription drugs than heterosexual young women (RR 1.29, 1.77 and 2.41, respectively).

A meta-analysis published in 2022, which included 105 studies, showed that the overall prevalence of alcohol consumption is higher in bisexual people than in lesbian or gay people and heterosexual people.[27]

(4) In this study, the definition of high-risk alcohol consumption meant consuming more than 14 drinks per week for men and more than 7 for women.

9.8. Weight, body image and eating behavior disorders

Younger people, as well as adults, who identify as LGB often experience discomfort with their bodies. Concern with the body and the importance of self-image are part of adolescence. However, this is a particularly vulnerable phase for risk situations, namely for eating behavior disorders. Some studies suggest that the risk of eating behavior disorders is increased in LGB youth.

A review published in 2018[28] showed that in most of the studies analyzed, individuals who identified as homosexual had an increased prevalence of restrictive diets, symptoms related to eating behavior disorders, compulsive behaviors towards food, and purging behaviors such as vomiting or laxative use. The differences found were more evident in men than in women. This review points out that the differences found are not only related to different sexual orientation, but also, and jointly, to ethnicity, race and other socioeconomic variables, drawing attention to the fact that risk determinants are multifactorial.

There has been an increased prevalence of overweight (body mass index (BMI) between 25 and 29.9 kg/m2) and obesity (BMI equal to or greater than 30 kg/m2) in lesbian women compared to heterosexual women. In a review published in 2014,[29] 37 studies mostly conducted in the United States were analyzed, with the vast majority of these concluding that the average BMI values and the percentage of women with a BMI equal to or greater than 30 kg/m2 is significantly higher in lesbian or bisexual women compared to heterosexual women.

Since there is, on the one hand, an increase in compulsive behaviors regarding food and, on the other hand, an increased prevalence of obesity and overweight in lesbian women compared to heterosexual women, it is important to assess whether the two factors are related to each other. A study published in 2016, which analyzed eating behavior and body weight in lesbian women, showed a statistically significant association between binge eating and obesity, with an OR of 2.73 (taking the group with normal BMI as a reference) and between binge eating and overweight, with an OR of 1.43. Other variables associated with obesity were rural residence, age and lower education.

A meta-analysis published in 2021 showed that there are eating behavior patterns more frequent in women with a certain type of sexual orientation, with heterosexual and bisexual women being those who present the greatest risks of eating behavior disorders.[30]

There is data that suggests that homosexual boys perceive their weight as being above normal even when this is not the case, and homosexual girls perceive their weight as normal or low when this does not correspond to reality.[31]

In general, it should be noted that eating behavior disorders, anorexia and bulimia, while being much more frequent in females, both in homosexual and heterosexual individuals, can have a significantly increased frequency in male homosexual individuals.

The issue of increased prevalence of obesity, especially in lesbian women, certainly has a multifactorial etiology which includes an movement of opposition and antagonism to heteronormative stereotypes, which we can characterize with the "Barbie" image, in which attractive women are tall and thin.

9.9. HIV infection in lesbian, gay or bisexual people

AIDS and HIV infection, in general, have been associated with the homosexual population. In the 1980s, AIDS was even called "the gay plague". Later, for many years, if not even to this day, when talking about HIV, one thinks of "risk groups" and these include homosexual people. In fact, the concept of risk group in relation to HIV infection has long been questioned and progressively abandoned, as it is understood that there are forms of transmission and risk behaviors for that same transmission, but pigeonholing people into risk groups is stigmatizing and discriminatory.

When thinking about sexual orientation and risk of HIV infection it is important to consider that the risk of transmission through sexual relations between two men is not comparable to the risk of transmission between two women.

For a long time it was assumed that there was no transmission of the HIV virus through woman-woman sexual relations,[32,33] with the CDC even publishing a report to this effect in 2006. However, there have been publications of cases of transmission in women who exclusively have sexual relations with women, with even epidemiological guidelines for this situation.[34,35,36,37] The hypotheses regarding the mode of transmission are that it happens when one of the women is infected and there is direct contact with blood, for example through digital penetration in situations where there may be small wounds on the fingers or through oral sex, or through small lesions on the vaginal wall and contact with shared sex toys.[38] However, the risk of transmission between women who have sexual relations exclusively with women is low.

On the contrary, in the European Union, the population of men who have sex with men (MSM) is currently the one that contributes the most to new cases of HIV infection. In 2016, 40% of new HIV infection diagnoses had MSM as the mode of transmission, with the second most frequent mode of transmission being sexual transmission in heterosexual people, responsible for 32% of new diagnoses.[39]

In the last decade, the incidence of HIV infections has decreased in women, heterosexual men and injecting drug users, but not in MSM. In addition to HIV infection, there also seems to be an increase, in this group, in the number of sexually transmitted infections, such as gonorrhea and syphilis.[40]

Considering the different transmission categories, the MSM category is the one with the lowest frequency of late presentation cases (38%) versus 58% when the transmission route was heterosexual sexual intercourse and 55% when the transmission route was injecting drug use. Late presentation is considered when the individual has, at the time of diagnosis, CD4 < 350/mm3. The fact that in the MSM group there are fewer cases of late presentation of the disease suggests that this subpopulation is more alert to the situation, seeking medical care earlier.[39]

Collecting a complete clinical history, including sexual history, described in detail in the previous chapter, is essential to anticipate risk situations and be able to act preventively.

HIV screening should be done by all people aged between 18 and 64 years. In the case of men who have sex with men (MSM) or women partners of MSM, screening should be repeated at least annually.[41]

Pre-exposure prophylaxis (PrEP) is recommended by the European AIDS Clinical Society for HIV-negative men who have casual sex with men, or sex with HIV-positive partners who are not on treatment, in situations where condoms are not used consistently. The use of PrEP provides a high level of protection against HIV infection but not against other sexually transmitted diseases.[42]

9.10. Other sexually transmitted infections in lesbian, gay or bisexual people

The LGB population, especially men who have sex with men without using condoms, has an increased risk for all sexually transmitted infections. Due to its frequency, Chlamydia infection stands out, both in men and women, and screening should be carried out annually in MSM.[43]

Chlamydia infection is often asymptomatic but can manifest in men as urethritis, epididymitis, or proctitis. In men who have sex with men (MSM) presenting with rectal symptoms, the possibility of lymphogranuloma venereum should be considered. In women, the infection can manifest as cervicitis, urethritis, pelvic inflammatory disease, or perihepatitis (Fitz-Hugh-Curtis syndrome).

Gonococcal infections, or gonorrhea, are also a very common sexually transmitted infection, especially in MSM. In women who have sex with women, the risk is unknown and seems to depend on sexual practices, namely digital penetration or penetration with sex toys, allowing infection through the transport of vaginal secretions.[48]

Like Chlamydia infections, Gonococcal infections can also be asymptomatic. The main disease presentations include, in men, urethritis, epididymitis, and proctitis. In women, it can manifest as urethritis, pelvic inflammatory disease, or cervicitis. Pharyngeal Gonococcal infections associated with oral sex, especially through contact of the penis with the oropharynx, are mostly asymptomatic. But they can manifest as pharyngitis.

Gonococcal infection can also have a systemic manifestation. In this infrequent situation, the condition may include purulent arthritis or the triad of tenosynovitis, dermatitis, and polyarthralgias. The condition is relatively serious and should be promptly treated as it can lead to destruction of the involved joints.

Bacterial vaginosis caused by anaerobic agents is relatively common in women who have sex with women, and seems to be directly associated with the number of sexual partners and the practice of oral sex.

Syphilis is a sexually transmitted infection that has been increasing in recent years, especially in young MSM. Syphilis has three stages of presentation: primary syphilis, with an isolated, usually asymptomatic skin lesion; secondary syphilis, which presents with maculopapular lesions on the soles of the feet and palms of the hands, skin lesions and lymphadenopathy; and tertiary syphilis, which can affect the heart or central nervous system. The association between syphilis and HIV infection is well known, so in the face of a syphilis diagnosis, laboratory tests for HIV are mandatory.

Hepatitis are infections that can be transmitted through sexual intercourse, either by transmission through semen or vaginal fluids or by transmission through blood, or even by fecal-oral transmission, as in the case of hepatitis A. Hepatitis C has been associated with HIV infection, especially in MSM.

HPV infection is detailed below in the chapters dedicated to cervical cancer and anal cancer.

9.11. Neoplasms in lesbian, gay or bisexual people

Analysis of the risk of neoplasms in LGB populations is limited by the lack of robust evidence on this topic. For some types of neoplasia, an increased prevalence has been described, related to sexual orientation, such as in breast cancer, cervical cancer or anal cancer.[44] The primary reason for this association is the existence of a high prevalence in LGB people of some of the known risk factors for each of these, and other, neoplasms. For example, LGB people have a higher prevalence of smoking, so it is reasonable to assume that they have an increased risk of lung cancer, even if this is exclusively due to tobacco.

Although it is important to distinguish what are directly associated risk factors, with biological plausibility, to a given neoplasm, from other factors that also have an association with that neoplasm, but via their relationship with other risk factors, this does not mean that this indirect association is not valuable.

If LGB people have an increased prevalence of risk factors associated with certain neoplasms, then they most likely also have an increased risk of those same neoplasms.[45] This is extremely important for the clinical evaluation of each person, since this information should condition the medical team to actively investigate and implement preventive measures against not only the risk factors, but also the oncological situations at higher risk.

Studies on lung cancer and colorectal cancer found no direct association between their prevalence and sexual orientation.[44] However, as LGB people have an increased prevalence of smoking and alcohol consumption, both risk factors for these neoplasms, screening and surveillance for these conditions should be performed regularly. Another aspect to consider is the association between HIV infection and risk of lung cancer.[46]

Endometrial cancer has been studied in lesbian women, comparing the risk with heterosexual women. The results are mixed, with a trend towards a possible increased risk in lesbian women, which was associated with nulliparity, obesity and much lower use of oral contraceptives.[47] At the same time, there are data pointing to a lower risk in women who have never had sexual intercourse with men.[48]

Data on prostate cancer in homosexual men are limited. Studies conducted[49] in the United States point to a lower prevalence of prostate cancer in homosexual men, 5.3% versus 16.5% in heterosexual men and 14.3% in bisexual men.[50] On the other hand, there seems to be an inverse relationship between HIV infection and risk of prostate cancer, with an estimated 50% risk reduction.[51]

As mentioned before in other topics, the fact that LGB people seek medical care less frequently can have important negative consequences with regard to screening and early detection of any type of cancer. In the specific case of prostate cancer, it is important to properly collect family history, identify other risk factors, such as smoking, and perform PSA according to the screening schemes recommended for the male population.

9.11.1. Breast cancer

Breast cancer is the most prevalent neoplastic condition in females and one of the greatest contributors to cancer mortality. It has been considered that breast cancer may have an increased prevalence in lesbian women, since they have a higher prevalence of risk factors associated with breast cancer compared to heterosexual women. Among these risk factors, nulliparity, obesity, alcohol consumption and smoking stand out, all of which are more frequent in lesbian women than in heterosexual women.[52] On the other hand, as previously mentioned, lesbian women are highly likely to have less access to preventive medical care, namely less breast cancer screening.[53]

Although there are very few studies that specifically evaluated the prevalence of breast cancer in lesbian women, a systematic review was published in 2013[54] that evaluated 15 studies. None of the identified studies evaluated incidence and the prevalence data are ambiguous, with studies showing higher prevalences in lesbian women compared to heterosexual women and others showing the opposite or finding no differences.

A study published in 2020 evaluated 58,378 women aged 40 or older, 2% of whom identified themselves as belonging to a sexual minority (lesbian or bisexual). In this study, the prevalence of breast cancer was similar between women belonging to sexual minorities and heterosexual women (4.7% vs. 5.0%, p = 0.67), and belonging to sexual minorities was not associated with the diagnosis of breast cancer.[55]

9.11. Neoplasms in lesbian, gay or bisexual people

Analysis of the risk of neoplasms in LGB populations is limited by the lack of robust evidence on this topic. For some types of neoplasia, an increased prevalence has been described, related to sexual orientation, such as in breast cancer, cervical cancer or anal cancer.[44] The primary reason for this association is the existence of a high prevalence in LGB people of some of the known risk factors for each of these, and other, neoplasms. For example, LGB people have a higher prevalence of smoking, so it is reasonable to assume that they have an increased risk of lung cancer, even if this is exclusively due to tobacco.

Although it is important to distinguish what are directly associated risk factors, with biological plausibility, to a given neoplasm, from other factors that also have an association with that neoplasm, but via their relationship with other risk factors, this does not mean that this indirect association is not valuable.

If LGB people have an increased prevalence of risk factors associated with certain neoplasms, then they most likely also have an increased risk of those same neoplasms.[45] This is extremely important for the clinical evaluation of each person, since this information should condition the medical team to actively investigate and implement preventive measures against not only the risk factors, but also the oncological situations at higher risk.

Studies on lung cancer and colorectal cancer found no direct association between their prevalence and sexual orientation.[44] However, as LGB people have an increased prevalence of smoking and alcohol consumption, both risk factors for these neoplasms, screening and surveillance for these conditions should be performed regularly. Another aspect to consider is the association between HIV infection and risk of lung cancer.[46]

Endometrial cancer has been studied in lesbian women, comparing the risk with heterosexual women. The results are mixed, with a trend towards a possible increased risk in lesbian women, which was associated with nulliparity, obesity and much lower use of oral contraceptives.[47] At the same time, there are data pointing to a lower risk in women who have never had sexual intercourse with men.[48]

Data on prostate cancer in homosexual men are limited. Studies conducted[49] in the United States point to a lower prevalence of prostate cancer in homosexual men, 5.3% versus 16.5% in heterosexual men and 14.3% in bisexual men.[50] On the other hand, there seems to be an inverse relationship between HIV infection and risk of prostate cancer, with an estimated 50% risk reduction.[51]

As mentioned before in other topics, the fact that LGB people seek medical care less frequently can have important negative consequences with regard to screening and early detection of any type of cancer. In the specific case of prostate cancer, it is important to properly collect family history, identify other risk factors, such as smoking, and perform PSA according to the screening schemes recommended for the male population.

9.11.1. Breast cancer

Breast cancer is the most prevalent neoplastic condition in females and one of the greatest contributors to cancer mortality. It has been considered that breast cancer may have an increased prevalence in lesbian women, since they have a higher prevalence of risk factors associated with breast cancer compared to heterosexual women. Among these risk factors, nulliparity, obesity, alcohol consumption and smoking stand out, all of which are more frequent in lesbian women than in heterosexual women.[52] On the other hand, as previously mentioned, lesbian women are highly likely to have less access to preventive medical care, namely less breast cancer screening.[53]

Although there are very few studies that specifically evaluated the prevalence of breast cancer in lesbian women, a systematic review was published in 2013[54] that evaluated 15 studies. None of the identified studies evaluated incidence and the prevalence data are ambiguous, with studies showing higher prevalences in lesbian women compared to heterosexual women and others showing the opposite or finding no differences.

A study published in 2020 evaluated 58,378 women aged 40 or older, 2% of whom identified themselves as belonging to a sexual minority (lesbian or bisexual). In this study, the prevalence of breast cancer was similar between women belonging to sexual minorities and heterosexual women (4.7% vs. 5.0%, $p = 0.67$), and belonging to sexual minorities was not associated with the diagnosis of breast cancer.[55]

9.11.2. Cervical Cancer

Cervical cancer is relatively common and is associated with human papillomavirus (HPV) infection, particularly HPV-16 and HPV-18. HPV infection occurs through sexual transmission. The risk of HPV infection in lesbian women was usually considered lower than that of heterosexual women, since sexually transmitted infections generally have a lower prevalence in women who have sex exclusively with women.[56] However, some studies have shown that the risk of STDs is not lower in lesbian women who have had sex with men. Moreover, lesbian women have a higher prevalence of other risk factors, such as tobacco use and obesity, which contribute to an increased risk of cervical cancer.[57]

One of the most effective ways to prevent cervical cancer is through HPV vaccination.

Screening through cervical cytology should be performed every 3 years in women between 21 and 65 years of age. It is important to consider, as mentioned earlier, that LGB individuals seek less medical care, so the possibility of not having adequate screening or vaccination increases.

9.11.3. Anal Cancer

Anal cancer is a relatively rare condition, but its prevalence has been increasing. Some studies show an increased incidence of anal neoplasia in men who have sex with men.[58] The incidence has been associated with the presence of HPV and HIV infection.[59] HPV is a sexually transmitted infection through contact with skin from the anogenital region, mucous membranes, or bodily fluids of an infected person.[60] There are numerous types of HPV, and their carcinogenic potential is substantially different. The subtypes associated with high carcinogenic risk include HPV-16, HPV-18, HPV-31, HPV-33, HPV-35, HPV-45, HPV-51, HPV-52, and HPV-

56.[61].Other risk factors for anal cancer include a high number of sexual partners, coexistence of sexually transmitted infections, smoking, and immunosuppression.

In a 2022 review that included 39 studies, the prevalence of anal cancer was 20% (95% CI, 17-29%), and ranged from 22% in men with HIV who have sex with men, to 13% in women and 12% in HIV-negative men who have sex with men. The sensitivity and specificity of cytology and HPV tests were 81% and 62% and 92% and 42%, respectively, and 93% and 33%, respectively for cytology and HPV co-testing.[62]

9.12. Mental illness and suicide

The LGB population is more likely, over their lifetime, to suffer from discrimination, family rejection, and even psychological and physical abuse, due to having a sexual orientation different from the majority of people. As with minorities in general, people are victims of ignorance, prejudice, and phobic behaviors. Exposure to this type of context and the anticipation that discrimination may occur translate into increased levels of stress, anxiety, and low self-esteem and self-confidence. It is therefore not surprising that the LGB population has a higher prevalence of mental illness, particularly mood disorders, including depression and anxiety.[63]

Depression showed an increased risk of about twice as high in the LGB population compared to the heterosexual population. The risk was not different in lesbian versus gay people. Studies that assessed anxiety show an increased risk compared to heterosexual people (RR 2.28), especially in gay and bisexual men.[64]

It is essential to always keep in mind the increased risk of mental disorders, especially depressive and anxiety disorders, in this population, being alert for signs and symptoms and anticipating the occurrence of more serious situations.

The results of a systematic review published in 2022 that included 21 studies and a total of 6,573 non-heterosexual and/or non-cisgender participants suggest that self-acceptance and self-compassion are significantly associated with mental health indicators in sexual and/or gender minority individuals, with a close relationship to internalized homophobia/ transphobia, especially in older adults and younger people with suicidal ideation. The results suggest that affirmative mental health care may benefit from promoting self-acceptance and self-compassion.[65]

Another study, also published in 2022, demonstrates the importance of safe community environments in promoting physical and mental health in sexual and/or gender minority people.[66]

The risk of suicide or suicidal ideation also appears to be increased in LGB people, especially younger ones. A meta-analysis published in 2017[67] analyzed LGB sexual orientation as a risk factor for suicide in adolescents. Of the studies analyzed, three[68,69,70] showed an association between sexual orientation and suicide risk, with increased risk in LGB people (OR 2.96 to 6.20 versus heterosexual people), and three other studies[71,72,73] showed no significant increase in risk between LGB and heterosexual groups. Overall, there was an increased risk of suicide in LGB youth compared to heterosexual youth, OR 2.32.

According to another review published in 2016[74] that included studies conducted in the United States, Canada, Europe, Australia, and New Zealand, the estimated lifetime prevalence of suicide attempts was 4% for heterosexual people and 11% to 20% for the LGB population.

Suicidal ideation was also more prevalent in LGB people of both genders compared to heterosexual people (RR 2.04).[64]

The main protective factors appear to be associated with family support specifically regarding sexual orientation and a supportive and inclusive climate from schools. Another important factor is establishing romantic relationships with same-sex partners, which allows the young lesbian or gay person to increase their self-esteem and, at the same time, seems to reduce levels of social stress.[75]

A meta-analysis published in 2022 evaluated suicidal ideation and suicide attempts in youth aged 12 to 25 belonging to sexual and/or gender minorities. The review included 44 studies. Overall, prejudice-based LGBTQIA+ victimization, general victimization, bullying, and negative family treatment were significantly associated with suicidal ideation and/or suicide attempts. In this review, discrimination and internalized homophobia and transphobia did not show a direct association with suicidal ideation and/or suicide attempts.[76]

A study conducted in European countries, published in 2020, compared suicidal ideation and suicide attempts in heterosexual and sexual minority adolescents. The prevalence of severe suicidal ideation was 5.1% in the heterosexual youth group and 12.7% in the sexual minority youth group (OR 2.72 (CI 1.54-4.80)). According to this study, European sexual minority youth are a high-risk group for suicide, regardless of objective factors such as victimization or substance abuse, confirming the need to develop primary and secondary preventive measures for sexual minority youth, including managing context vulnerabilities and stressors, and context-oriented interventions should focus on social and economic factors, as well as the potentially different risk profile between genders.[77]

9.13. Other pathologies with increased prevalence in lesbian, gay, or bisexual people

9.13.1. Cardiovascular risk and disease

Although cardiovascular risk appears to be increased in LGB people compared to heterosexual people, studies have not found significant differences regarding cardiovascular disease (CVD).

In addition to the data presented above regarding a higher prevalence of smoking, a higher prevalence of alcohol consumption, and a higher prevalence of overweight and obesity in LGB people, there also seems to be a higher prevalence of insulin resistance, hypertension, and sedentariness. Together, these factors mean that the risk of CVD is higher in the LGB population compared to the analogous heterosexual population. However, studies that analyzed CVD did not find differences between LGB and heterosexual people.[78,79]

In 2020, the American Heart Association published a document for the first time aimed at assessing cardiovascular health in sexual and/or gender minority populations. In this document, it assumes that there is growing evidence that lesbian, gay, bisexual, transgender, or queer (LGBTQ) people experience disparities among several cardiovascular risk factors compared to heterosexual and cisgender people. These disparities mainly result from exposure to psychosocial stressors throughout life. In this document, the American Heart Association reviews the existing literature on cardiovascular health in LGBTQ adults. Despite the identified methodological limitations, there is evidence that LGBTQ adults (particularly lesbian, bisexual, and transgender women) experience cardiovascular health disparities. More research, including studies with longitudinal designs, will be needed to elucidate physiological mechanisms, assess social and clinical determinants of cardiovascular health, and identify potential targets for behavioral interventions. Furthermore, according to this document, LGBTQ health content should be integrated into health profession curricula and continuing education to ensure a multifaceted approach that integrates best practices in health promotion and cardiovascular care for this population.[80]

9.13.2. Sleep quality and duration

Sleep disorders are associated with decreased quality of life, increased prevalence of chronic disease, and even mortality. Until relatively recently, sleep pathology was studied individually, with population-level studies being relatively recent. These studies have been demonstrating that there is an association between economically or socially disadvantaged or minority population groups and sleep disorders or changes in sleep patterns. In this context, it can be assumed that homosexual people may constitute a risk group for sleep pathology, given that they are a group with high levels of stress and anxiety and, in some situations, with unfavorable social, family, and economic contexts.

A study published in 2017[81] that included 68,960 people residing in the United States evaluated sleep characteristics and associated pathology in people with different sexual orientations. In this study, the percentage of heterosexual people who slept less than 6 hours per day was 8.7% versus 11.2% in homosexual and bisexual people. The percentage of people who reported feeling "little rested" was 36.2% in the heterosexual population versus 43.5% and 44.8% in the homosexual and bisexual population, respectively. Regarding the percentage of people who reported "difficulty falling asleep" and "waking up at night", an increased prevalence was also found in the homosexual and bisexual population.

The results obtained in this study were controlled for other sociodemographic variables and physical and mental health status. When sleep data were analyzed in models controlled for the remaining variables, there was no direct association between sexual orientation and sleep duration, but this association remained with regard to "feeling little rested" (OR 1.20, homosexual people versus heterosexual people) and "difficulty falling asleep" (OR 1.24, homosexual people versus heterosexual people; OR 1.38, bisexual people versus heterosexual people). Furthermore, when analyzing people based not only on their sexual orientation but also on gender, it was found that the aforementioned differences are specific to the female homosexual and bisexual population, using the male heterosexual population as a reference. Other studies have confirmed these results,[82,83,84,85] and have shown that female and male homosexual populations have higher consumption of drugs for sleep induction and maintenance.[86]

9.13.3. Asthma

The prevalence of asthma seems to be increased in lesbian or bisexual women. A meta-analysis published in 2018[87] analyzed 12 studies that compared the prevalence of asthma in lesbian, bisexual women or women who had sexual relations with other women, and six of them found significantly increased values of asthma prevalence compared to heterosexual women. One of the studies, published in 2014,[88] describes an asthma prevalence of 15.3% in heterosexual women versus 22.2% in lesbian women and 26.4% in bisexual women. Another study,[89] published in the same year, points to values of 13.7% in heterosexual women versus 20.8% and 21.5% in lesbian and bisexual women, respectively.

The reason for the increased prevalence of asthma in lesbian and bisexual women is unclear. Some factors that may be associated are the increased prevalence of obesity and overweight and high levels of stress. Once again, we are most likely facing a theme in which Intersectionality prevails, that is, each individual is affected by multiple factors and circumstances that as a whole contribute to an increase in prevalence, in this case, of asthma.[90]

9.13.4. Gynecological diseases

Although there is a belief that some gynecological diseases, namely Polycystic Ovary Syndrome (PCOS), are more frequent in lesbian women than in heterosexual women, this was not verified in a meta-analysis published in 2017.[91] Although some studies have concluded that the frequency of PCOS was increased in the lesbian and bisexual population, the aggregate result of several studies showed no significant difference compared to the heterosexual population. Similarly, no differences were found between groups with regard to the frequency of endometriosis. In bisexual women, a higher frequency of chronic pelvic pain was found when compared to the frequency in heterosexual women.

Bibliography

[1] Damaskos P., Amaya B., Gordon R., Walters C. B. Intersectionality and the LGBT Cancer Patient. InSeminars in oncology nursing. 2018 Jan 8. W. B. Saunders.

[2] Ryan C., Huebner D., Diaz R. M., Sanchez J. Family rejection as a predictor of negative health outcomes in white and Latino lesbian, gay, and bisexual young adults. Pediatrics.

2009 Jan 1; 123(1): 346-52.

[3] Human Rights Campaign Growing up LGBT in America. 2012. Retrieved from http://www.hrc.org//files/assets/resources/Growing-Up-LGBT-in-America_Report.pdf [Accessed in 20/4/18].

[4] Lei n.º 2/2016. Diário da República, 1.ª série – N.º 41 – 29 de fevereiro de 2016. https://dre.pt//application/conteudo/73740375 [Accessed in 20/4/18].

[5] Lei n.º 17/2016. Diário da República, 1.ª série – N.º 116 – 20 de junho de 2016. https://dre.pt//application/conteudo/74738646. [Accessed in 20/4/18].

[6] Lei n.º 25/2016. Diário da República, 1.ª série – N.º 160 – 22 de agosto de 2016. https:///dre.pt/application/conteudo/75177806. [Accessed in 20/4/18].

[7] Lei n.º 90/2021. Diário da República, 1.ª série – N.º 242 – 16 de dezembro de 2021. https:///files.dre.pt/1s/2021/12/24200/0001300016.pdf [Accessed in 17/11/22].

[8] De Sutter P., Dutré T. I., Meerschaut F. V., Stuyver I. S., Van Maele G. E., Dhont M. A.PCOS in lesbian and heterosexual women treated with artificial donor insemination. Reproductive biomedicine online. 2008 Jan 1; 17(3): 398-402.

[9] Nordqvist S., Sydsjö G., Lampic C., Åkerud H., Elenis E., Skoog Svanberg A. Sexual orientation of women does not affect outcome of fertility treatment with donated sperm.Human Reproduction. 2014 Jan 15; 29(4): 704-11.

[10] Hodson K., Meads C., Bewley S. Lesbian and bisexual women's likelihood of becoming pregnant: a systematic review and meta-analysis. BJOG: An International Journal of Obstetrics & Gynaecology. 2017 Feb 1; 124(3): 393-402.

[11] Crowl A., Ahn S., Baker J. A meta-analysis of developmental outcomes for children of samesex and heterosexual parents. Journal of GLBT Family Studies. 2008 Aug 12; 4(3): 385-407.

[12] Bos H. M., Knox J. R., Van Rijn-van Gelderen L., Gartrell N. K. Same-sex and different-sex parent households and child health outcomes: Findings

from the National Survey of Children's Health. Journal of Developmental & Behavioral Pediatrics. 2016 Apr 1; 37(3): 179-87.

[13] Kabir Z., Keogan S., Clarke V., Clancy L. Second-hand smoke exposure levels and tobacco consumption patterns among a lesbian, gay, bisexual and transgender community in Ireland. Public Health. 2013 May 1; 127(5): 467-72.

[14] Lindström M., Axelsson J., Modén B., Rosvall M. Sexual orientation, social capital and daily tobacco smoking: a population-based study. BMC public health. 2014 Dec; 14(1): 565.

[15] McCabe S. E., Matthews A. K., Lee J. G., Veliz P., Hughes T. L., Boyd C. J. Tobacco Use and Sexual Orientation in a National Cross-sectional Study: Age, Race/Ethnicity, and Sexual Identity – Attraction Differences. American journal of preventive medicine. 2018 Apr 12.

[16] Blosnich J., Lee J. G., Horn K. A systematic review of the aetiology of tobacco disparities for sexual minorities. Tobacco control. 2013 Mar 1; 22(2): 66-73.

[17] Rosario M., Schrimshaw E. W., Hunter J. Predictors of substance use over time among gay, lesbian, and bisexual youths: an examination of three hypotheses. Addict Behav. 2004; 29: 1623e31.

[18] McKirnan D. J., Tolou-Shams M., Turner L., et al. Elevated risk for tobacco use among men who have sex with men is mediated by demographic and psychosocial variables. Subst Use Misuse. 2006; 41: 1197e208.

[19] Hughes T. L., Johnson T. P., Matthews A. K. Sexual orientation and smoking: results from a multisite women's health study. Subst Use Misuse. 2008; 43: 1218e39.

[20] Mays V. M., Cochran S. D. Mental health correlates of perceived discrimination among lesbian, gay, and bisexual adults in the United States. Am J Public Health. 2001; 91: 1869e76.

[21] Willoughby B. L. B., Doty N. D., Malik N. M. Victimization, family rejection, and outcomes of gay, lesbian, and bisexual young people: The role of negative GLB identity. Journal of GLBT Family Studies. 2010; 6: 403e24.

[22] Shokoohi, M., Salway, T., Ahn, B., & Ross, L. E. (2021). Disparities in the prevalence of cigarette smoking among bisexual people: a systematic

review, meta-analysis and metaregression. Tobacco control, 30(e2), e78-e86. https://doi.org/10.1136/tobaccocontrol-2020--055747.

[23] Green K. E., Feinstein B. A. Substance use in lesbian, gay, and bisexual populations: An update on empirical research and implications for treatment. Psychology of Addictive Behaviors. 2012 Jun; 26(2): 265.

[24] Bränström R., Pachankis J. E. Sexual orientation disparities in the co-occurrence of substance use and psychological distress: a national population-based study (2008-2015).

Social psychiatry and psychiatric epidemiology. 2018 Apr 1; 53(4): 403-12.

[25] Gonzales G., Przedworski J., Henning-Smith C. Comparison of health and health risk factors between lesbian, gay, and bisexual adults and heterosexual adults in the United States: results from the National Health Interview Survey. JAMA internal medicine. 2016 Sep 1; 176(9): 1344-51.

[26] Caputi T. L. Sex and orientation identity matter in the substance use behaviors of sexual minority adolescents in the United States. Drug & Alcohol Dependence. 2018 Mar 7.

[27] Shokoohi, M., Kinitz, D. J., Pinto, D., Andrade-Romo, Z., Zeng, Z., Abramovich, A., Salway, T., & Ross, L. E. (2022). Disparities in alcohol use and heavy episodic drinking among bisexual people: A systematic review, meta-analysis, and meta-regression. Drug and alcohol dependence, 235, 109433. https://doi.org/10.1016/j.drugalcdep.2022.109433.

[28] Calzo J. P., Blashill A. J., Brown T. A., Argenal R. L. Eating disorders and disordered weight and shape control behaviors in sexual minority populations. Current psychiatry reports. 2017 Aug 1; 19(8): 49.

[29] Eliason M. J., Ingraham N., Fogel S. C., et al.: A systematic review of the literature on weight in sexual minority women. Womens Health Issues. 2015; 25: 162-175.

[30] Dotan, A., Bachner-Melman, R., & Dahlenburg, S. C. (2021). Sexual orientation and disordered eating in women: a meta-analysis. Eating and weight disorders: EWD, 26(1), 13-25. https://doi.org/10.1007/s40519-019-00824-3.

[31] Hadland S. E., Austin S. B., Goodenow C. S., Calzo J. P. Weight misperception and unhealthy weight control behaviors among sexual minorities in the general adolescent population. Journal of Adolescent Health. 2014 Mar 1; 54(3): 296-303.

[32] Fethers K., Marks C., Mindel A., Estcourt C. S. Sexually transmitted infections and risk behaviours in women who have sex with women. Sexually Transmitted Infections. 2000 Oct 1; 76(5): 345-9.

[33] Petersen L. R., Doll L., White C., Chu S. No evidence for female-to-female HIV transmission among 960,000 female blood donors. The HIV Blood Donor Study Group. Journal of acquired immune deficiency syndromes. 1992; 5(9): 853-5.

[34] Kwakwa H. A., Ghobrial M. W. Female-to-female transmission of human immunodeficiency virus. Clinical Infectious Diseases. 2003 Feb 1; 36(3): e40-1.

[35] Bezerra, A. L. L., Sorensen, W., Rodrigues, T. B., Sousa, S. M. L., Carneiro, M. S., Polaro, S. H. I., Ramos, A. M. P. C., Ferreira, G. R. O. N., Gir, E., Reis, R. K., & Botelho, E. P.

(2022). HIV epidemic among Brazilian women who have sex with women: An ecological study. Frontiers in public health, 10, 926560. https://doi.org/10.3389/fpubh.2022.926560.

[36] Molin, S. B., De Blasio, B. F., & Olsen, A. O. (2016). Is the risk for sexually transmissible infections (STI) lower among women with exclusively female sexual partners compared with women with male partners? A retrospective study based on attendees at a Norwegian STI clinic from 2004 to 2014. Sexual health, 13(3), 257-264. https://doi.org/10.1071/SH15193.

[37] Muzny, C. A., Harbison, H. S., Pembleton, E. S., & Austin, E. L. (2013). Sexual behaviors, perception of sexually transmitted infection risk, and practice of safe sex among southern African American women who have sex with women. Sexually transmitted diseases, 40(5), 395-400.

[38] Deol A. K., Heath-Toby A. HIV risk for lesbians, bisexuals & other women who have sex with women. Gay Men's Health Crisis. June. 2009.

[39] European Centre for Disease Prevention and Control/WHO Regional Office for Europe. HIV/AIDS surveillance in Europe 2017 – 2016 data. Stockholm: ECDC; 2017.

[40] European Commission. Review of HIV and sexually transmitted infections among men who have sex with men (MSM) in Europe. Berlin, Germany. ESTICOM; 2017

[41] Norma n.º 058/2011, atualizada em 10 de dezembro de 2014, Direção-Geral da Saúde – Diagnóstico e Rastreio Laboratorial da Infeção pelo Vírus da Imunodeficiência Humana (VIH) – http://www.pnvihsida.dgs.pt/informacao-tecnica-e-cientifica111/legislacao-em-vigor//norma-n-0582011-atualizada-em-10-de-dezembro-de-2014-direcao-geral-da-saude.aspx [Accessed in 21/4/18].

[42] EACS Guidelines 2017. European AIDS Clinical Society (EACS). http://www.pnvihsida.dgs.pt//informacao-tecnica-e-cientifica111/recomendacoes-internacionais/normas-eacs11.aspx [Accessed in 20/4/18].

[43] Wood S. M., Salas-Humara C., Dowshen N. L. Human immunodeficiency virus, other sexually transmitted infections, and sexual and reproductive health in lesbian, gay, bisexual, transgender youth. Pediatric Clinics. 2016 Dec 1; 63(6): 1027-55.

[44] Quinn G. P., Sanchez J. A., Sutton S. K., Vadaparampil S. T., Nguyen G. T., Green B. L., Kanetsky P. A., Schabath M. B. Cancer and lesbian, gay, bisexual, transgender/transsexual, and queer/questioning (LGBTQ) populations. CA: a cancer journal for clinicians. 2015 Sep 1; 65(5): 384-400.

[45] Wakefield D. (2021). Cancer care disparities in the LGBT community. Current opinion in supportive and palliative care, 15(3), 174-179. https://doi.org/10.1097/SPC.00000000000- 00557.

[46] Hou W., Fu J., Ge Y., Du J., Hua S. Incidence and risk of lung cancer in HIV-infected patients. J Cancer Res Clin Oncol. 2013; 139(11): 1781-1794.

[47] Zaritsky E., Dibble S. L. Risk factors for reproductive and breast cancers among older lesbians. J Womens Health (Larchmt) 2010; 19(1): 125-131.

[48] Valanis B. G., Bowen D. J., Bassford T., Whitlock E., Charney P., Carter R. A. Sexual orientation and health: comparisons in the women's health initiative sample. Arch Fam Med. 2000; 9(9): 843-853

[49] Blank T. O. Gay men and prostate cancer: invisible diversity. J Clin Oncol. 2005; 23(12): 2593-2596.

[50] Boehmer U., Miao X., Ozonoff A. Cancer survivorship and sexual orientation. Cancer. 2011; 117(16): 3796-3804.

[51] Shiels M. S., Goedert J. J., Moore R. D., Platz E. A., Engels E. A. Reduced risk of prostate cancer in U.S. Men with AIDS. Cancer Epidemiol Biomarkers Prev. 2010; 19(11): 2910-2915.

[52] Graham R., Berkowitz B., Blum R., Bockting W., Bradford J., de Vries B., Garofalo R., Herek G., Howell E., Kasprzyk D., Makadon H. The health of lesbian, gay, bisexual, and transgender people: Building a foundation for better understanding. Washington, DC: Institute of Medicine. 2011 Mar 31.

[53] Hart S. L., Bowen D. J. Sexual orientation and intentions to obtain breast cancer screening. J Womens Health (Larchmt) 2009; 18(2): 177-185.

[54] Meads C., Moore D. Breast cancer in lesbians and bisexual women: systematic review of incidence, prevalence and risk studies. BMC public health. 2013 Dec; 13(1): 1127.

[55] Williams, A. D., Bleicher, R. J., & Ciocca, R. M. (2020). Breast Cancer Risk, Screening, and Prevalence Among Sexual Minority Women: An Analysis of the National Health Interview Survey. LGBT health, 7(2), 109-118. https://doi.org/10.1089/lgbt.2019.0274.

[56] Molin S. B., De Blasio B. F., Olsen A. O. Is the risk for sexually transmissible infections (STI) lower among women with exclusively female sexual partners compared with women with male partners? A retrospective study based on attendees at a Norwegian STI clinic from 2004 to 2014. Sexual health. 2016 Jun; 13(3): 257-64.

[57] Waterman L., Voss J. HPV, cervical cancer risks, and barriers to care for lesbian women. Nurse Pract. 2015; 40(1): 46-53.

[58] Machalek D. A., Poynten M., Jin F., et al. Anal human papillomavirus infection and associated neoplastic lesions in men who have sex with men: a systematic review and meta-analysis. Lancet Oncol. 2012; 13(5): 487-500.

[59] Dunne E. F., Nielson C. M., Stone K. M., Markowitz L. E., Giuliano A. R. Prevalence of HPV infection among men: A systematic review of the literature. J Infect Dis. 2006; 194(8): 1044-1057.

[60] Giuliano A. R., Nyitray A. G., Kreimer A. R., et al. EUROGIN 2014 roadmap: Differences in human papillomavirus infection natural history, transmission and human papillomavirusrelated cancer incidence by gender and anatomic site of infection. International Journal of Cancer. 2014

[61] Bravo I. G., Felez-Sanchez M. Papillomaviruses: Viral evolution, cancer and evolutionary medicine. Evolution, medicine, and public health. 2015; 2015(1): 32-51.

[62] Clarke, M. A., Deshmukh, A. A., Suk, R., Roberts, J., Gilson, R., Jay, N., Stier, E. A., & Wentzensen, N. (2022). A systematic review and meta-analysis of cytology and HPV-related biomarkers for anal cancer screening among different risk groups. International journal of cancer, 151(11), 1889-1901. https://doi.org/10.1002/ijc.34199.

[63] Chakraborty A., McManus S., Brugha T. S., Bebbington P., King M. Mental health of the non-heterosexual population of England. The British journal of psychiatry. 2011 Feb 1; 198(2): 143-8.

[64] King M., Semlyen J., Tai S. S., Killaspy H., Osborn D., Popelyuk D., Nazareth I. A systematic review of mental disorder, suicide, and deliberate self harm in lesbian, gay and bisexual people. BMC psychiatry. 2008 Dec; 8(1): 70.

[65] Carvalho, S. A., & Guiomar, R. (2022). Self-Compassion and Mental Health in Sexual and Gender Minority People: A Systematic Review and Meta-Analysis. LGBT health, 9(5), 287-302. https://doi.org/10.1089/lgbt.2021.0434.

[66] Flentje, A., Clark, K. D., Cicero, E., Capriotti, M. R., Lubensky, M. E., Sauceda, J., Neilands, T. B., Lunn, M. R., & Obedin-Maliver, J. (2022). Minority Stress, Structural Stigma, and Physical Health Among Sexual and Gender Minority Individuals: Examining the Relative Strength of the Relationships. Annals of behavioral medicine: a publication of the Society of Behavioral Medicine, 56(6), 573-591. https://doi.org/10.1093/abm/kaab051.

[67] Miranda-Mendizábal A., Castellví P., Parés-Badell O., Almenara J., Alonso I., Blasco M. J., Cebrià A., Gabilondo A., Gili M., Lagares C., Piqueras J. A. Sexual orientation and suicidal behaviour in adolescents and young adults: systematic review and meta-analysis. The British Journal of Psychiatry. 2017 Mar 2: bjp-p.

[68] Fergusson D. M., Horwood L. J., Beautrais A. L. Is sexual orientation related to mental health problems and suicidality in young people? Arch Gen Psychiatry. 1999; 56: 876-80.

[69] Silenzio V. M. B., Pena J. B., Duberstein P. R., Cerel J., Knox K. L. Sexual orientation and risk factors for suicidal ideation and suicide attempts among adolescents and young adults. Am J Public Health. 2007; 97: 2017-9.

[70] Whitlock J., Muehlenkamp J., Eckenrode J., Purington A., Baral Abrams G., Barreira P., et al. Nonsuicidal self-injury as a gateway to suicide in young adults. J Adolesc Health. 2013; 52: 486-92.

[71] Bearman P. S., Moody J. Suicide and friendships among American adolescents. Am J Public Health. 2004; 94: 89-95.

[72] Young R., Riordan V., Stark C. Perinatal and psychosocial circumstances associated with risk of attempted suicide, non-suicidal self-injury and psychiatric service use. A longitudinal study of young people. BMC Public Health. 2011; 11: 875.

[73] Fried L. E., Williams S., Cabral H., Hacker K. Differences in risk factors for suicide attempts among 9th and 11th grade youth: a longitudinal perspective. J Sch Nurs. 2012; 29: 113-22.

[74] Hottes T. S., Bogaert L., Rhodes A. E., Brennan D. J., Gesink D. Lifetime prevalence of suicide attempts among sexual minority adults by study sampling strategies: a systematic review and meta-analysis. American journal of public health. 2016 May; 106(5): e1-2.

[75] Russell S. T., Fish J. N. Mental health in lesbian, gay, bisexual, and transgender (LGBT) youth. Annual review of clinical psychology. 2016 Mar 28; 12: 465-87.

[76] de Lange, J., Baams, L., van Bergen, D. D., Bos, H. M. W., & Bosker, R. J. (2022). Minority Stress and Suicidal Ideation and Suicide Attempts

Among LGBT Adolescents and Young Adults: A Meta-Analysis. LGBT health, 9(4), 222-237. https://doi.org/10.1089/lgbt.2021.0106.

[77] Gambadauro, P., Carli, V., Wasserman, D., Balazs, J., Sarchiapone, M., & Hadlaczky, G. (2020). Serious and persistent suicidality among European sexual minority youth. PloS one, 15(10), e0240840. https://doi.org/10.1371/journal.pone.0240840.

[78] Caceres B. A., Brody A., Luscombe R. E., Primiano J. E., Marusca P., Sitts E. M., Chyun D. A systematic review of cardiovascular disease in sexual minorities. American journal of public health. 2017 Apr; 107(4): e13-21.

[79] Meads C., Martin A., Grierson J., Varney J. Systematic review and meta-analysis of diabetes mellitus, cardiovascular and respiratory condition epidemiology in sexual minority women. BMJ open. 2018 Apr 1; 8(4): e020776.

[80] Caceres, B. A., Streed, C. G., Jr, Corliss, H. L., Lloyd-Jones, D. M., Matthews, P. A., Mukherjee, M., Poteat, T., Rosendale, N., Ross, L. M., & American Heart Association Council on Cardiovascular and Stroke Nursing; Council on Hypertension; Council on Lifestyle and Cardiometabolic Health; Council on Peripheral Vascular Disease; and Stroke Council (2020). Assessing and Addressing Cardiovascular Health in LGBTQ Adults: A Scientific Statement From the American Heart Association. Circulation, 142(19), e321-e332. https://doi.org/

/10.1161/CIR.0000000000000914.

[81] Chen J. H., Shiu C. S. Sexual orientation and sleep in the US: a National Profile. American journal of preventive medicine. 2017 Apr 1; 52(4): 433-42.

[82] Fricke J., Sironi M. Dimensions of sexual orientation and sleep disturbance among young adults. Preventive medicine reports. 2017 Dec 1; 8: 18-24.

[83] Li P., Huang Y., Guo L., Wang W., Xi C., Lei Y., Luo M., Pan S., Deng X., Zhang W. H., Lu C. Is sexual minority status associated with poor sleep quality among adolescents? Analysis of a national cross-sectional survey in Chinese adolescents. BMJ open. 2017 Dec 1; 7(12): e017067.

[84] Dai H., Hao J. Sleep Deprivation and Chronic Health Conditions Among Sexual Minority Adults. Behavioral sleep medicine. 2017 Jul 23: 1-5.

[85] Caceres, B. A., & Hickey, K. T. (2020). Examining Sleep Duration and Sleep Health Among Sexual Minority and Heterosexual Adults: Findings From NHANES (2005-2014). Behavioral sleep medicine, 18(3), 345-357. https://doi.org/10.1080/15402002.2019.1591410.

[86] Galinsky A. M., Ward B. W., Joestl S. S., Dahlhamer J. M. Sleep duration, sleep quality,and sexual orientation: findings from the 2013-2015 National Health Interview Survey. Sleep health. 2018 Feb 1; 4(1): 56-62.

[87] Meads C., Martin A., Grierson J., Varney J. Systematic review and meta-analysis of diabetes mellitus, cardiovascular and respiratory condition epidemiology in sexual minority women. BMJ open. 2018 Apr 1; 8(4): e020776.

[88] Boehmer U., Miao X., Linkletter C., Clark M. A. Health conditions in younger, middle, and older ages: are there differences by sexual orientation? LGBT health. 2014 Sep 1; 1(3): 168-76.

[89] Blosnich J. R., Lee J. G., Bossarte R., Silenzio V. M. Asthma disparities and within-group differences in a national, probability sample of same-sex partnered adults. American journal of public health. 2013 Sep; 103(9): e83-7.

[90] Talham, C. J., Montiel Ishino, F. A., & Williams, F. (2022). A Socioecological Mixture Model of Asthma Prevalence Among Sexual Minority Adults in the United States. LGBT health, 10.1089/lgbt.2021.0338. Advance online publication. https://doi.org/10.1089/lgbt.2021.0338.

[91] Robinson K., Galloway K. Y., Bewley S., Meads C. Lesbian and bisexual women's gynaecological conditions: a systematic review and exploratory meta-analysis. BJOG: An International Journal of Obstetrics & Gynaecology. 2017 Feb 1; 124(3): 381-92.

Ana Macedo

Chapter 10 - Health specificities in transgender people

10.1. Clinical history and physical examination in transgender people

The collection of clinical history and physical examination in transgender people is essentially similar to the collection of clinical history in any other person. However, there are some specificities, of an emotional, social and physical nature that are important to take into consideration.

In most situations, transgender people feel more vulnerable to health professionals than the general population. It is the responsibility of health professionals and organizations to minimize this possible discomfort and promote inclusive environments that provide confidence and security, enabling a holistic clinical approach that is truly person-centered.

10.1.1. Collecting clinical history in transgender people

The name and the way of addressing a transgender person is in itself one of the situations to take into account, as previously mentioned. When someone addresses a person, they use the grammatical gender of the names, pronouns or adjectives that correspond to the gender of their name, registered on identification cards and/or, if they are seeing or hearing the person in question, to the gender that corresponds to the physical appearance and voice.

In transgender people, the name assigned to them at birth, which coincided with the gender designated at that time, does not correspond to the gender with which the person identifies. This aspect is particularly important when a child or young person who expresses a gender identity different from that of their name is addressed by a name "non-coincident with gender".

It is not uncommon for a transgender person, with a gender expression that does not correspond to the sex and gender assigned to them at birth, to still have in their documents and identification the name of birth registration, although in their daily life they use another name. In this situation there is a mismatch between the gender expression and the name registered in the identification documents, which may from the outset, even before any clinical intervention, create situations of discomfort that may compromise the entire therapeutic relationship.

It is recommended that in health services, when any person registers administratively, they are asked by what name they want to be addressed, regardless of the name that is registered on the identification card and the person's appearance. The health team must respect the name and gender with which the person identifies, using the corresponding grammatical forms throughout the consultation. If at any time, by mistake, they don't do it, this fact should not be overlooked, and the best attitude is to make the incident explicit and apologize, continuing the consultation.

In the medical approach, the collection of clinical history should include gender identity directly, although it should not focus too much on this aspect. The person who goes to a health service has a reason for going to the consultation (or the emergency room) and this should be explored first. After collecting information about the reason for consultation (emergency) and data on the current situation, the previous history including the history related to gender identity should be explored. In this topic, it should be addressed whether the person is undergoing, or has undergone, medical and/or surgical therapy for gender affirmation. In the case of hormonal treatment, it is important to know what drugs are being used, at what doses and for how long, and whether these were prescribed by medical professionals or if the person self-medicated.

Knowledge of hormonal therapy is essential as it has potential adverse effects, drug interactions, is associated with an increased risk of some pathologies and determines a different evaluation against reference values for laboratory tests (see description below).

The evaluation of previous gender affirmation surgeries is fundamental, not only to allow exploring any risk or complication of the surgery itself, but also to plan, for example, cancer screening. For example, in a transgender male person, it is necessary to consider performing cervical or ovarian cancer screening, depending on whether or not a hysterectomy and oophorectomy have been performed.

If the reason for consultation is directly related to the issue of gender identity, for example a person who seeks their family doctor for the first time to address the topic, the history should be collected in as much detail as possible, assessing the person's expectations regarding the future, namely regarding the performance of hormonal therapy and gender affirmation surgery. The person should be referred to a specialty consultation.

It is important to bear in mind that, if taking a sexual history always raises issues with some degree of sensitivity, in the case of transgender people the topic is even more delicate. Thus, history taking should be planned in order to use inclusive language, not make any kind of judgment regarding sexual behaviors and practices, asking questions openly and not directing the answer either in the sense of corresponding to the "socially acceptable", or in the sense of meeting possible stereotypes or prejudices. Sexual orientation and sexual behavior do not depend on gender identity and as such it is not permissible to make assumptions in this domain based on gender identity or expression.

The use of gender-neutral language in relation to possible sexual partners is important for anyone, but in the case of transgender people it is even more so. Another important aspect is to ask if the person has questions or doubts regarding sexual behaviors, regardless of whether they have experienced them or not.

Sexual orientation, in transgender or cisgender people, does not in itself allow us to anticipate types of higher or lower risk sexual behavior. That is, for example, a person who identifies as heterosexual does not exclude the possibility of practicing anal sex. According to data from a study conducted in the United States, 44% of men and 36% of women who identify as heterosexual said they had practiced anal sex on at least one occasion.

In addition to questions regarding sexual behaviors, it is important to assess and ask clearly and directly if there are signs or symptoms of sexually transmitted diseases.

It should be taken into consideration that pregnancy can occur in transgender men who have not undergone hysterectomy and salpingo-oophorectomy, and the topic should be addressed when collecting clinical history.

Discomfort in approaching sexual history, either on the part of doctors or on the part of the transgender person, make this topic little or not explored in most consultations, contributing to increase the risk of STDs and neoplastic diseases, due to insufficient screening evaluation care.

Transgender people have an increased risk of some mental health disorders. Thus, in the clinical history, symptoms characteristic of mood disorders, anxiety and depression, including suicidal ideation, should be proactively addressed.

Family history, especially in its social-familial dimension, is relevant since transgender people often suffer from social and/or family isolation and discrimination. Knowledge of the surrounding social support context is crucial to anticipate possible risk situations.

10.1.2. Physical examination of the transgender person

Regardless of the person's gender identity, the physical examination should focus on the current medical history and be directed towards the complaints and symptoms. In some situations, transgender people may feel more discomfort than a cisgender person regarding body exposure, and the physical examination may be perceived as traumatic. To minimize possible discomfort in the situation, it is particularly important to reflect on the medical need to assess sensitive areas such as the thoracic region or the pelvic area, in an emergency or first consultation. Another relevant aspect is to inform the person about all the evaluations that will be carried out, that is, to say at each moment "I will touch...", "you will feel pressure on...".

With time and increased confidence, the person will feel more comfortable exposing their body, allowing for a more complete physical examination and enabling a favorable context for transmitting information about it, in terms of health promotion and risk analysis.

Before proceeding with a detailed physical examination, it is essential to have knowledge of the medical history, especially regarding medical and surgical gender affirmation treatments.

When assessing the pelvic area, sometimes difficulties arise about the best nomenclature to use for describing the external sexual organs. The simplest way to deal with the situation is to always ask the person which term they prefer. For example, a transgender man may not feel comfortable with a reference to "his vagina" and may prefer the area to be identified more vaguely as "in your pelvic area".

On physical examination, transgender people undergoing hormonal therapy present secondary sexual characteristics of the female or male gender, more or less marked, depending on the prescribed therapy, its duration, and serum levels of estrogens and testosterone. Thus, in transgender men undergoing hormonal treatment, one can expect facial and body hair growth, increased muscle mass and redistribution of body fat, androgenetic alopecia, acne, vaginal atrophy, and clitoral hypertrophy. In transgender women undergoing hormonal treatment, one can expect to find breast development and increased breast volume, reduced muscle mass and redistribution of body fat, absence of facial hair, thin skin, and reduced testicular volume.

In transgender people who have undergone gender affirmation surgeries, the physical examination depends on the type of surgery performed (see gender affirmation surgeries chapter). For example, in a transgender woman who has undergone vaginoplasty surgery, the created neovagina is anatomically different, usually having a more posterior orientation and, being a blind pouch, without a cervix. Knowledge of the situation will allow for a better approach in the gynecological examination.

The pelvic examination of a transgender man is usually associated with great anxiety. However, this examination and the performance of a cervical cytology smear are essential to enable adequate surveillance of cervical cancer risk.

10.2. Laboratory tests in transgender people

Many laboratory parameters, complete blood count, biochemistry and other tests have reference values assigned according to sex. To date, the available evidence on how reference values for laboratory parameters should be defined and interpreted in transgender people undergoing or who have undergone medical and/or surgical treatment for gender affirmation is very limited. In this context, the intervals of normal values for each test should be interpreted cautiously, taking into account the hormonal levels (estrogens and testosterone) of each individual.[1,2]

10.2.1. Complete blood count in transgender people

Studies conducted in transgender women have shown a significant reduction in erythropoiesis. A study published in 2018[3] evaluated 21 transgender women undergoing hormonal treatment with oral estrogens, having shown a reduction of about 5% in hematocrit, reduction in hemoglobin and red blood cell count, compared to the values before gender affirmation treatment. This reduction is mainly attributed to the reduction in serum testosterone, and not to the increase in estradiol. At the same time, the globular volume did not show variation, nor did the white blood cell count, the leukocyte formula or the platelet count. In contrast, in the eleven transgender men included, undergoing hormonal treatment with intramuscular testosterone, there was an increase in red blood cell count, hemoglobin level and hematocrit.

A study published in 2014[4] included 55 transgender women undergoing hormonal therapy for gender affirmation for at least 6 months, having compared the results of several laboratory parameters with those obtained in two control groups of healthy female and male individuals. The hematocrit and hemoglobin values of transgender women were similar to those of the female control group and significantly lower than those of the male control group.

The values found suggest that in situations of transgender people undergoing hormonal therapy and with the respective estrogen or testosterone values within the target values, the laboratory values currently defined for women and men can be considered, respectively for transgender women or men. Or use as reference values for hemoglobin and hematocrit, in the case of transgender women, the lower values of the lower limit of normal for females and the upper values of the upper limit of normal for males.[7,5]

10.2.2. Lipid profile in transgender people

The variation in lipid profile in transgender individuals undergoing hormonal treatment for gender affirmation has been studied by several authors, and the results are not completely concordant. Two meta-analyses performed, one in 2010[6] and another in 2017,[7] showed an increase in triglycerides in both transgender groups and a reduction in HDL in transgender men. In the remaining lipid parameters, no significant changes were detected. Given that the magnitude of the differences found is relatively small, their clinical significance is questionable, especially with regard to the need to change primary prevention measures.

10.3. Smoking in transgender people

Tobacco in combination with estrogen therapy leads to an increased risk of venous thromboembolism (VTE). Thus, all transgender women undergoing estrogen hormone therapy should be strongly advised not to smoke and warned about the risk of VTE.

Smoking per se is not an absolute contraindication for estrogen therapy. In situations where people are unable or unwilling to quit smoking, an attempt should be made to reduce the smoking load, and the possibility of transdermal estrogen therapy instead of oral therapy should be considered, as well as the use of preventive treatments such as the administration of antiplatelet agents. However, there is no robust evidence on the risk-benefit ratio of the latter option.[7]

10.4. Body weight and fat mass in transgender people

Gender affirmation hormone therapy results in a change in body weight and composition. As these variables are associated with cardiovascular risk, it is important to understand the estimated effects in both transgender women and men.

In transgender women, hormone treatment leads to an increase in weight, an increase in fat mass, and a decrease in lean mass. In transgender men, there is an increase in body weight, a decrease in fat mass, and an increase in lean mass. These changes are consistent with an increased cardiovascular risk in transgender women.[8] In transgender women there is an increase in hip circumference, while the opposite situation occurs in transgender men.[9]

10.5. Cardiovascular risk in transgender people

Various diseases, particularly cardiovascular and cerebrovascular diseases, have a risk of occurrence that is related to sex. The pathophysiological basis for this relationship is mainly due to hormonal differences and the physical and mental changes they cause. In this context, it is important to evaluate how the risk is established in transgender populations undergoing gender-affirming hormone therapy and/or who have undergone gender-affirming surgeries.

The available evidence suggests that the cardiovascular risk of transgender men treated with testosterone is similar to that of cisgender women. The evidence regarding transgender women is less robust. Studies conducted have shown an increased morbidity and mortality from acute myocardial infarction and stroke compared to the cisgender male population. However, the results of these studies were not adjusted for other risk factors such as smoking, obesity, and diabetes.

Several studies show that transgender women have higher prevalences of smoking, obesity, diabetes, and dyslipidemia, and lower levels of physical activity,[10] so the increased risk of cardiovascular and cerebrovascular disease may be due not to hormonal changes but rather to the presence of other risk factors.

Cardiovascular risk calculation tables and equations are based on sex. To date, there are no specific tables for transgender people. Thus, the recommendations are to calculate the cardiovascular risk of transgender people using the general tables and considering the sex designated at birth or the gender with which the person identifies and expresses, depending on the duration of exposure to gender-affirming hormones (estrogens, antiandrogens or testosterone).[7,11]

10.6. Bone density and osteoporosis in transgender people

The impact of long-term treatment with gender-affirming hormones on bone metabolism remains unknown. A meta-analysis conducted in 2017,[12] which evaluated 639 transgender individuals, assessed bone mineral density before starting hormone treatment and after 12 and 24 months, concluding that in transgender women there is an increase in lumbar spine bone density. However, the results are not homogeneous. Some studies conclude that there is an increase in osteoporosis in transgender women, associated with the presence of other known risk factors for osteoporosis such as low level of physical activity, reduced muscle mass, and low levels of vitamin D.[13,14]

The risk of osteoporosis is also associated with insufficient doses of estrogen therapy.

In transgender men, most studies have not shown significant changes in bone density.

In 2019, the International Society for Clinical Densitometry (ISCD) published guidelines on the topic specifically referring to transgender people.

This document advocates the following:

Performing bone densitometry (DXA) in transgender individuals if they have any of the following conditions:

History of gonadectomy or therapy that reduces endogenous levels of gonadal steroids before starting hormone therapy.

Hypogonadism in people who will not initiate gender-affirming hormone therapy.

Use of glucocorticoids or hyperparathyroidism.

Low bone density.

Individuals undergoing treatment to suppress puberty, such as GnRH analogues.

Non-adherence or inadequate doses of gender-affirming hormone therapy.

Plan to discontinue gender-affirming hormone therapy.

Presence of other risks of bone loss or fragility fracture.

- The intervals for performing bone densitometry should be individualized based on the clinical situation: typically every 1-2 years until bone density stabilizes or improves, after which the intervals can be extended.
- Calculation of T- and Z-scores in transgender individuals:

T-scores should be calculated using a uniform Caucasian female normative database (not race-adjusted) for all transgender individuals of all ethnic groups; it is recommended to use a T-score of < - 2.5 or less for the diagnosis of osteoporosis in all transgender individuals age 50 or older, regardless of hormonal status.

Calculate Z-scores using the normative database that matches the individual's gender identity.

If requested, Z-scores can also be calculated using the normative database corresponding to the sex designated at birth.

For non-binary individuals, the normative database corresponding to the sex designated at birth should be used.

Gender data should be obtained from the admission questionnaire.

The parameters to be included in the DXA report for transgender individuals are the same as those included in reports for the general population, but when specially requested, the report should include Z-scores calculated according to both male and female databases.[15]

10.7. Pelvic pain in transgender men

Pelvic pain is a relatively common condition in transgender men and poses challenges in differential diagnosis. Clinical history is a fundamental element in this context, and should be exhaustive and assess in detail the onset of pain, duration, relieving and aggravating factors, intensity, and irradiation. In addition to characterizing the pain, it is important to detail previous pathology, gynecological history, and gender-affirming therapy and/or surgeries. Sexual history is also an important piece of data since certain types of sexual behavior may constitute risk factors.[16]

Etiologies are diverse and include, among others, atrophic or infectious vaginitis, cervicitis, pelvic inflammatory disease, cystitis, endometriosis, post-surgical adhesions, sexually transmitted diseases, ovarian cyst torsion or rupture, appendicitis, intestinal pathology, musculoskeletal or neurogenic pathology. In addition to these etiologies, the possibility of traumatic injury in the context of accident or violence should be evaluated.[7]

In individuals who have not undergone hysterectomy and/or salpingo-oophorectomy and who have vaginal penetrative sex with a male partner (with viable sperm), pregnancy and ectopic pregnancy should be investigated.

The physical examination should be performed but it should be anticipated that it may be anxiety-provoking and even traumatic for the person. Thus, as mentioned above, all procedures should be explained, trying to put the person in the most comfortable position possible. The objective examination should include abdominal inspection, percussion, and palpation. If possible, and with the person's consent, a gynecological examination should be performed.

10.8. Abnormal uterine bleeding in transgender men

In transgender men of childbearing age who choose not to undergo hysterectomy and oophorectomy or receive gender-affirming hormone therapy, regular menstrual cycles are expected to continue.

In individuals receiving testosterone hormone therapy at physiological doses, amenorrhea usually occurs within about 6 months. Testosterone causes ovarian suppression and endometrial atrophy. However, the time to amenorrhea depends not only on the dose, frequency, and route of administration of testosterone, but also on any previous pathology. Individuals with irregular menstrual cycles prior to starting hormone therapy may have underlying pathology and this may be the cause of persistent menstrual cycles even after months of testosterone administration.[7]

Abnormal uterine bleeding is considered to be that which persists after 6 to 12 months of testosterone therapy in individuals with testosterone levels within the target range for the male gender and with suppression of LH and FSH.[17]

The etiology of abnormal uterine bleeding is diverse and includes endometrial polyps, adenomyosis, leiomyomatosis, endometrial hyperplasia, uterine neoplasia, pregnancy, coagulopathy, ovarian dysfunction, and iatrogenic causes.

10.9. Testicular pain

Pain in the scrotal region is a condition whose prevalence remains unknown but is reported by some transgender women. The main cause associated with this pain is the (voluntary) positioning of the testicles inside the inguinal canal, a practice followed by some individuals with the aim of obtaining a feminine visual appearance. This practice is accompanied by the positioning of the penis and scrotal skin between the legs, longitudinally, towards the anus. The position of the genitals is maintained by tight underwear or the use of adhesive materials.

Regular use of this practice, understood as a form of gender affirmation, can result in traumatic, mechanical or neuropathic pain, but also inguinal hernia, urinary reflux, prostatitis, orchitis or cystitis.[7]

Although this is the most frequent cause of testicular pain, other etiologies such as neoplasms, hernias, hydrocele, torsion, infection, or trauma should be evaluated.

10.10. HIV infection and other sexually transmitted diseases

The prevalence of HIV infection in transgender women was estimated at 19.1%, based on a meta-analysis published in 2017,[18] which included 11,066 transgender women from 39 studies conducted in 15 countries. Analysis of studies conducted in European countries, the United States, and Australia points to prevalence values of 21.6%.

Prevalence of 19.9% (95% CI 14.7% - 25.1%) for transgender females (n = 48,604) and 2.56% (95% CI 0.0%-5.9%) for transgender males (n = 6460). The overall OR for HIV infection, compared to individuals over 15 years old, was 66.0 (95% CI 51.4-84.8) for transgender females and 6.8 (95% CI 3.6-13.1) for transgender males.[19]

One of the reasons that may underlie the high risk of HIV infection in transgender females is related to the risk associated with certain sexual behaviors. Some studies show that transgender females who have sex with cisgender men more often assume a passive role in anal sex, when compared to cisgender men who have sex with other cisgender men.[20] Furthermore, transgender females also reported using condoms less frequently and having a greater number of sexual partners. On the other hand, the risk of HIV infection in cisgender men who have sex with transgender women also appears to be higher than that of the cisgender male population in general.[21]

It is important to consider that one of the main forms of infection transmission occurs through unprotected anal sex, with the highest probability of transmission associated with the passive or receptive position.[22]

The risk of HIV transmission through neovaginal penetrative sex after vaginoplasty remains unknown.

With regard to transgender males, the risk is substantially lower. However, several studies have been reporting that this risk is higher than previously assumed.[23,24] The main route of transmission in transgender males is similar to that described for transgender females and MSM, that is, transmission occurs through unprotected sex, especially anal sex.[18]

It is assumed that the transgender population has an increased vulnerability to the risk of HIV infection, not only due to the possibility of sexual transmission in the contexts described above and in heterosexual relationships, but also because this subpopulation has a higher prevalence of addictive behaviors and negative psychosocial factors that in themselves increase vulnerability to communicable diseases.[25]

The prevention, screening and treatment of HIV infection in transgender people is similar to that recommended for the general population. Although the available evidence is limited, since estrogen metabolism occurs through the P450 enzyme system, it is expected that there may be interactions between estrogen therapy and antiretroviral therapy (ART), without however compromising the safety and effectiveness of these treatments.[26]

The evaluation and diagnosis of HIV infection depends, first of all, on considering this clinical possibility in any person. In the case of transgender people, especially transgender females, the risk of disease is increased, so it should be taken into account through careful collection of medical and sexual history and laboratory evaluation.

The risk of HIV in transgender people does not depend on gender identity but rather on sexual behaviors, or others, associated with an increased risk of the disease. Collecting a detailed sexual history is important for risk assessment and prevention optimization (see previous chapter Clinical history and physical examination in LGB people).

As mentioned previously, HIV testing should be performed by all people between the ages of 18 and 64. In the case of transgender people, and assuming that, overall, they have an increased risk of HIV transmission, annual screening is recommended.

Pre-exposure prophylaxis (PrEP) is indicated by the European AIDS Clinical Society in situations of increased risk, such as unprotected sex with

HIV-infected partners or situations in which HIV-negative transgender people who have casual sex with men, in situations where condoms are not used consistently. The use of PrEP provides a high level of protection against HIV infection, but not against other sexually transmitted diseases.[42]

The risk and manifestations of other sexually transmitted diseases in transgender people is fundamentally associated with their sexual orientation and especially their sexual practices. This topic is addressed in more detail in a previous subchapter with the same designation, within the chapter Specificities in health in the LGB population.

10.11. Mental illness and suicide in transgender people

Depression is a very prevalent condition and has a greatly increased frequency in transgender people. As mentioned regarding LGB people, the fact that they are exposed to high levels of stress, sometimes referred to as minority stress, discrimination, lack of family and social support, as well as low self-esteem, are in themselves risk factors for depression.

In the case of transgender people, the levels of discrimination and psychological and physical violence are higher than those of LGB people and create a favorable context for the occurrence of mood disorders, namely depression and anxiety. At the same time, the feeling of discomfort with the body and low self-esteem, which is present in most people before starting gender affirmation therapies, further increases the risk of depression.[27] Some studies comparing the frequency of depression in transgender people before and during or after gender affirmation therapies show that depression is more frequent before starting gender affirmation therapy.[28,29]

Anxiety, in general, is more prevalent in transgender people than in cisgender people,[30] with an estimated 70% of transgender people having or developing a mood or anxiety disorder throughout their lives. The risk factors seem to overlap with those described for depression. Regarding anxiety, it is important to try to specify and diagnose the type of anxiety. For example, generalized anxiety (presence of excessive anxiety and worry about various issues, events and activities) is a different situation from social anxiety (characterized by disproportionate fear or anxiety when a person is and interacts with other people, for a period of at least 6 months) and should be treated specifically.

A study conducted in Europe in 2004[31] points to a prevalence of social anxiety of 6.8% and a prevalence of specific phobias of 8.7%. In another review[32] the prevalence of these situations in transgender populations was estimated at 11% and 25%, respectively. Panic disorder was estimated at 2.7% in the general population and 13.1% in the transgender population. In this study, the most frequent disorders were specific phobia (25%), panic disorder (13%) and social phobia (11%) in transgender males and specific phobia (17%), social phobia (10%) and obsessive-compulsive disorder (OCD) (10%) in transgender females. Overall, the studies found a higher prevalence of anxiety in transgender males than in transgender females.

The same review states that the prevalence of anxiety is higher in transgender people who have not undergone gender affirmation therapy. The body changes obtained through hormonal therapy and/or surgeries lead to an increase in self-esteem and self-confidence and better quality of life,[33,34] which presents itself as a protective factor for mental illness.

Many studies have evaluated the prevalence of suicide, suicidal ideation and self-mutilation in transgender people, concluding that this group has an increased risk for each of these situations, although the results have some variation. A review carried out in 2016,[35] which included 31 studies conducted in Europe, the United States, Australia and Canada, reports a lifetime prevalence of self-mutilation that varies between 19% and 38%, being higher in younger people. The prevalence of suicide attempt varied among the different studies, with values between 10% and 42%. A meta-analysis published in 2017[36] points to a prevalence of suicidal ideation of 51.7% in transgender females and 45.4% in transgender males. The prevalence of suicide attempt was similar in both groups, 31% and 32%, respectively.

Bibliography

[1] Cheung, A. S., Lim, H. Y., Cook, T., Zwickl, S., Ginger, A., Chiang, C., & Zajac, J. D. (2021). Approach to Interpreting Common Laboratory Pathology Tests in Transgender Individuals. The Journal of clinical endocrinology and metabolism, 106(3), 893-901. https://doi.org/10.1210/clinem/dgaa546.

[2] Irwig M. S. (2021). Which reference range should we use for transgender and gender diverse patients? The Journal of clinical endocrinology and metabolism, 106(3), e1479-e1480. https://doi.org/10.1210/clinem/dgaa671.

[3] Vita R., Settineri S., Liotta M., Benvenga S., Trimarchi F. Changes in hormonal and metabolic parameters in transgender subjects on cross-sex hormone therapy: A cohort study. Maturitas. 2018 Jan 1; 107: 92-6.

[4] Roberts T. K., Kraft C. S., French D., Ji W., Wu A. H., Tangpricha V., Fantz C. R. Interpreting laboratory results in transgender patients on hormone therapy. The American journal of medicine. 2014 Feb 1; 127(2): 159-62.

[5] Greene, D. N., McPherson, G. W., Rongitsch, J., Imborek, K. L., Schmidt, R. L., Humble, R. M., Nisly, N., Dole, N. J., Dane, S. K., Frerichs, J., & Krasowski, M. D. (2019). Hematology reference intervals for transgender adults on stable hormone therapy. Clinica chimica acta; international journal of clinical chemistry, 492, 84-90. https://doi.org/10.1016/j.cca.2019.02.011.

[6] Elamin M. B., Garcia M. Z., Murad M. H., Erwin P. J., Montori V. M. Effect of sex steroid use on cardiovascular risk in transsexual individuals: a systematic review and meta-analyses. Clin Endocrinol (Oxf). 2010 Jan; 72(1): 1-10.

[7] Maraka S., Singh Ospina N., Rodriguez-Gutierrez R., Davidge-Pitts C. J., Nippoldt T. B., Prokop L. J., Murad M. H. Sex steroids and cardiovascular outcomes in transgender individuals: a systematic review and meta-analysis. The Journal of Clinical Endocrinology & Metabolism. 2017 Sep 13; 102(11): 3914-23.

[8] Klaver M., Dekker M. J., Mutsert R., Twisk J. W., Heijer M. Cross-sex hormone therapy in transgender persons affects total body weight, body fat and lean body mass: a meta-analysis. Andrologia. 2017 Jun 1; 49(5).

[9] Klaver, M., de Blok, C. J. M., Wiepjes, C. M., Nota, N. M., Dekker, M. J., de Mutsert, R., Schreiner, T., Fisher, A. D., T'Sjoen, G. and Den Heijer, M., 2018. Changes in regional body fat, lean body mass and body shape in trans persons using cross-sex hormonal therapy: results from a multicenter prospective study. European journal of endocrinology, 178(2), pp.165-173.

[10] Wierckx K., Elaut E., Declercq E., Heylens G., De Cuypere G., Taes Y., et al. Prevalence of cardiovascular disease and cancer during cross-sex hormone therapy in a large cohort of trans persons: a case-control study. Eur J Endocrinol Eur Fed Endocr Soc. 2013 Oct; 169(4): 471-8.

[11] Aranda, G., Halperin, I., Gomez-Gil, E., Hanzu, F. A., Seguí, N., Guillamon, A., & Mora, M. (2021). Cardiovascular Risk Associated With Gender Affirming Hormone Therapy in Transgender Population. Frontiers in endocrinology, 12, 718200. https://doi.org/10.3389/ /fendo.2021.718200.

[12] Singh-Ospina N., Maraka S., Rodriguez-Gutierrez R., Davidge-Pitts C., Nippoldt T. B., Prokop L. J., Murad M. H. Effect of sex steroids on the bone health of transgender individuals: a systematic review and meta-analysis. The Journal of Clinical Endocrinology & Metabolism. 2017 Sep 13; 102(11): 3904-13.

[13] Van Caenegem E., Taes Y., Wierckx K., Vandewalle S., Toye K., Kaufman J-M, et al. Low bone mass is prevalent in male-to-female transsexual persons before the start of crosssex hormonal therapy and gonadectomy. Bone. 2013 May; 54(1): 92-7.

[14] Wierckx K., Mueller S., Weyers S., Van Caenegem E., Roef G., Heylens G., et al. Longterm evaluation of cross-sex hormone treatment in transsexual persons. J Sex Med. 2012 Oct1; 9(10): 2641-51.

[15] Shuhart, C. R., Yeap, S. S., Anderson, P. A., Jankowski, L. G., Lewiecki, E. M., Morse, L. R., Rosen, H. N., Weber, D. R., Zemel, B. S., & Shepherd, J. A. (2019). Executive Summary of the 2019 ISCD Position Development Conference on Monitoring Treatment, DXA Cross-calibration and Least Significant Change, Spinal Cord Injury, Peri-prosthetic and Orthopedic Bone Health, Transgender Medicine, and Pediatrics. Journal of clinical densitometry: the official journal of the International Society for Clinical Densitometry,22(4), 453-471. https://doi.org/10.1016/j.jocd.2019.07.001.

[16] Jarrell J. F., Vilos G. A., Allaire C., Burgess S., Fortin C., Gerwin R., et al. Consensus guidelines for the management of chronic pelvic pain. J Obstet Gynaecol Can JOGC J Obstétrique Gynécologie Can JOGC. 2005 Aug; 27(8): 781-826.

[17] Munro M. G., Critchley H. O. D., Broder M. S., Fraser I. S., FIGO Working Group on Menstrual Disorders. FIGO classification system (PALM-COEIN) for causes of abnormal uterine bleeding in nongravid women of reproductive age. Int J Gynaecol Obstet Off Organ Int Fed Gynaecol Obstet. 2011 Apr; 113(1): 3-13.

[18] Baral S. D., Poteat T., Strömdahl S., Wirtz A. L., Guadamuz T. E., Beyrer C. Worldwide burden of HIV in transgender women: a systematic review and meta-analysis. The Lancet infectious diseases. 2013 Mar 1; 13(3): 214-22.

[19] Stutterheim, S. E., van Dijk, M., Wang, H., & Jonas, K. J. (2021). The worldwide burden of HIV in transgender individuals: An updated systematic review and meta-analysis. PloS one, 16(12), e0260063. https://doi.org/10.1371/journal.pone.0260063.

[20] Salazar L. F., Crosby R. A., Jones J., Kota K., Hill B., Masyn K. E. Contextual, experiential, and behavioral risk factors associated with HIV status: a descriptive analysis of transgender women residing in Atlanta, Georgia. Int J STD AIDS. 2017; 0(0): 1-8.

[21] Gamarel K. E., Reisner S. L., Darbes L. A., Hoff C. C., Chakravarty D., Nemoto T., et al. Dyadic dynamics of HIV risk among transgender women and their primary male sexual partners: the role of sexual agreement types and motivations. AIDS Care. 2016; 28(1): 104-11.

[22] Baggaley R. F., White R. G., Boily M. C. HIV transmission risk through anal intercourse: systematic review, meta-analysis and implications for HIV prevention. Int J Epidemiol. 2010; 39: 1048-63.

[23] Rowniak S., Chesla C., Rose C. D., Holzemer W. L. Transmen: the HIV risk of gay identity. AIDS Educ Prev. 2011; 23: 508-20.

[24] Stephens S. C., Bernstein K. T., Philip S. S. Male to female and female to male transgender persons have different sexual risk behaviors yet similar rates of STDs and HIV. AIDS Behav. 2011; 15: 683-86.

[25] Poteat T., Malik M., Scheim A., Elliott A. HIV Prevention Among Transgender Populations: Knowledge Gaps and Evidence for Action. Current HIV/AIDS Reports. 2017 Aug 1; 14(4): 141-52.

[26] Radix A., Sevelius J., Deutsch M. B. Transgender women, hormonal therapy and HIV treatment: a comprehensive review of the literature and recommendations for best practices. Journal of the International AIDS Society. 2016; 19(3Suppl 2).

[27] Witcomb G. L., Bouman W. P., Claes L., Brewin N., Crawford J. R., Arcelus J. Levels of depression in transgender people and its predictors:

Results of a large matched control study with transgender people accessing clinical services. Journal of affective disorders. 2018 Aug 1; 235: 308-15.

[28] Costa R., Colizzi M. The effect of cross-sex hormonal treatment on gender dysphoria individuals' mental health: a systematic review. Neuropsychiatric disease and treatment. 2016; 12: 1953.

[29] Colizzi M., Costa R., Todarello O. Transsexual patients' psychiatric comorbidity and positive effect of cross-sex hormonal treatment on mental health: results from a longitudinal study. Psychoneuroendocrinology. 2014 Jan 1; 39: 65-73.

[30] Heylens G., Elaut E., Kreukels B. P., Paap M. C., Cerwenka S., Richter-Appelt H., Cohen- Kettenis P. T., Haraldsen I. R., De Cuypere G. Psychiatric characteristics in transsexual individuals: multicentre study in four European countries. The British Journal of Psychiatry. 2014 Feb 1; 204(2): 151-6.

[31] Alonso J., Angermeyer M. C., Bernert S., Bruffaerts R., Brugha T. S., Bryson H., Girolamo G. D., Graaf R. D., Demyttenaere K., Gasquet I., Haro J. M. Prevalence of mental disorders in Europe: results from the European Study of the Epidemiology of Mental Disorders (ESEMeD) project. Acta psychiatrica scandinavica. 2004 Jun 1; 109(s420): 21-7.

[32] Millet N., Longworth J., Arcelus J. Prevalence of anxiety symptoms and disorders in the transgender population: A systematic review of the literature. International Journal of Transgenderism. 2017 Jan 2; 18(1): 27-38.

[33] Colizzi M., Costa R., Pace V., Todarello O. Hormonal treatment reduces psychobiological distress in gender identity disorder, independently of the attachment style. The journal of sexual medicine. 2013 Dec 1; 10(12): 3049-58.

[34] Colizzi M., Costa R., Todarello O. Transsexual patients' psychiatric comorbidity and positive effect of cross-sex hormonal treatment on mental health: results from a longitudinal study. Psychoneuroendocrinology. 2014 Jan 1; 39: 65-73.

[35] Marshall E., Claes L., Bouman W. P., Witcomb G. L., Arcelus J. Non-suicidal self-injury and suicidality in trans people: a systematic review of the literature. International review of psychiatry. 2016 Jan 2; 28(1): 58-69.

[36] Adams N., Hitomi M., Moody C. Varied reports of adult transgender suicidality: synthesizing and describing the peer-reviewed and gray literature. Transgender health. 2017 Apr 1; 2(1): 60-75.

[37] Labanca, T., Mañero, I., & Pannunzio, M. (2020). Transgender patients: considerations for routine gynecologic care and cancer screening. International journal of gynecological cancer: official journal of the International Gynecological Cancer Society, 30(12), 1990-1996. https://doi.org/10.1136/ijgc-2020-001860.

[38] Sonnenblick E. B., Shah A. D., Goldstein Z., Reisman T. Breast Imaging of Transgender Individuals: A Review. Current Radiology Reports. 2018 Jan 1; 6(1): 1.

[39] Kiely D. Transgender Patient Screening: Breast Cancer Risk Assessment and Screening Recommendations. Clinical journal of oncology nursing. 2017 Jun; 21(3): E67-70.

[40] Braun H., Nash R., Tangpricha V., Brockman J., Ward K., Goodman M. Cancer in transgender people: evidence and methodological considerations. Epidemiologic reviews. 2017 Jan 1; 39(1): 93-107.

[41] Trum H. W., Hoebeke P., Gooren L. J. Sex reassignment of transsexual people from a gynecologist's and urologist's perspective. Acta Obstet Gynecol Scand. 2015 Jun; 94(6): 563-7.

[42] Cebula H., Pham T. Q., Boyer P., et al. Regression of meningiomas after discontinuation of cyproterone acetate in a transsexual patient. Acta Neurochir (Wien). 2010; 152(11): 1955-1956

[43] Elbers J. M., Giltay E. J., Teerlink T., Scheffer P. G., Asscheman H., Seidell J. C., et al. Effectsof sex steroids on components of the insulin resistance syndrome in transsexual subjects. Clin Endocrinol (Oxf). 2003; 58(5): 562-71.

[44] Moverley, J., Loebner, S., Carmona, B., & Vuu, D. (2021). Considerations for Transgender People With Diabetes. Clinical diabetes: a publication of the American Diabetes Association, 39(4), 389–396. https://doi.org/10.2337/cd21-0011.

[45] Connelly, P. J., Marie Freel, E., Perry, C., Ewan, J., Touyz, R. M., Currie, G., & Delles, C. (2019). Gender-Affirming Hormone Therapy,

Vascular Health and Cardiovascular Disease in Transgender Adults. Hypertension (Dallas, Tex.: 1979), 74(6), 1266-1274. https://doi.org/ /10.1161/HYPERTENSIONAHA.119.13080.

[46] Elamin M. B., Garcia M. Z., Murad M. H., Erwin P. J., Montori V. M. Effect of sex steroid use on cardiovascular risk in transsexual individuals: A systematic review and meta-analyses. Clinical endocrinology. 2010 Jan 1; 72(1): 1-0.

[47] Wierckx K., Mueller S., Weyers S., Van Caenegem E., Roef G., Heylens G., T'sjoen G. Long-term evaluation of cross-sex hormone treatment in transsexual persons. The journal of sexual medicine. 2012 Oct 1; 9(10): 2641-51.

Glossary

Agender (adjective) - A person who defines themselves as not having a gender or having a neutral gender. It is a form of non-binary gender identity.

Asexual (adjective) - A person with a total, partial, or conditional absence of sexual attraction to any person, regardless of their biological sex or gender.

Bisexual (adjective) - A person who has romantic feelings, physical attraction, or sexual attraction to both people of their own gender and people of the opposite gender.

Gender affirmation surgeries - Surgical procedures that aim to modify the body so that it conforms to the gender identity with which the person identifies.

Cisgender (adjective) - People who identify with the gender and sex assigned to them at birth. People who are not transgender.

Coming out - The first time a person reveals their sexual orientation to someone, identifying as lesbian, gay, or bisexual. Or the first time a person reveals their gender identity to someone and identifies as transgender.

Sexual behavior - Specific behavior that involves sexual activity. It is often used to define risk assessment patterns for some diseases. In this context (of behavior), it can be said that an individual has sexual partners of the same sex and/or the opposite sex, but one cannot directly infer whether they are heterosexual, homosexual, bisexual, pansexual or asexual.

Gender dysphoria - A DSM-5 diagnosis given to people whose gender identity does not correspond to the sex and gender assigned at birth.

Gender spectrum - Classification that considers gender to be established on a continuum between feminine and masculine, being able to assume any position. It is opposed to a binary gender classification in which there is only feminine and masculine.

Gender expression - The way a person expresses (shows) their gender to the outside world (to other people). Gender expression includes, for example, clothing, haircut, accessories or gestures. Gender expression usually coincides with gender identity and may or may not correspond to the sex and gender assigned at birth.

Gay (adjective) - A boy or man (cisgender or transgender) who has romantic feelings, physical attraction, or sexual attraction to people of his own gender, that is, to boys or men (cisgender or transgender). The term is sometimes used as a synonym for homosexual, and can be applied to people of both genders.

Gender - Gender refers to social, cultural, psychological and behavioral characteristics associated with the feminine and the masculine. In each society, the models are different but give rise to cultural, social and individual expressions that define the feminine and the masculine.

Binary gender - Considers two unique categories for gender, feminine and masculine.

Fluid gender - A person who does not identify with a single gender. Identifies or expresses an unfixed gender, through a gender spectrum.

Non-binary gender - People who do not identify as either feminine or masculine, regardless of the sex and gender assigned to them at birth. They may identify as neutral gender, both genders, a combination of the two, or have a fluid gender.

Neutral gender - People who identify with a non-binary gender, in a position on the gender spectrum equidistant from masculine and feminine.

Heteronormative - Designates that heterosexuality is the norm and assumes that people are heterosexual.

Heterosexual (adjective) - A person who has romantic feelings, physical attraction, or sexual attraction to people of the opposite gender.

Homosexual (adjective) - A person who has romantic feelings, physical attraction, or sexual attraction to people of their own gender.

Gender identity - The individual's innate feeling of belonging to the feminine gender, masculine gender, neither of these, or both. Gender identity may or may not coincide with the sex and gender designated at birth.

Gender incongruence (sometimes used as a synonym for gender dysphoria) - Situations in which the gender identity does not coincide with the sex and gender assigned at birth and that cause discomfort and stress to the individual.

Lesbian (adjective) - A girl or woman (cisgender or transgender) who has romantic feelings, physical attraction, or sexual attraction to people of her own gender, that is, to girls or women (cisgender or transgender).

Sexual and/or gender minority - A group whose gender identity and/or sexual orientation differ from those of the majority of people in the society in which they are inserted.

Gender non-conformity - Manifestations of the individual of a certain gender (assigned at birth) that do not correspond to the cultural norm of expression of that gender or to the typical role or behavior. For example, choice of toys, clothes or colors.

Sexual orientation - Identification between the gender of the individual and the gender of the people to whom they are physically, emotionally and sexually attracted.

Pansexual (adjective) - A person who has romantic feelings, physical attraction, or sexual attraction to both people of their own gender and people of another gender. Similar term to bisexual, but does not assume a binary gender identity.

Queergender (adjective) - A person who does not identify with the defined categories for sex and gender. Assumes several unfixed positions along the gender spectrum.

Sex assigned (or attributed) at birth - Biological sex, usually assigned according to the anatomy of the external genital organs and, if available, the karyotype.

Transgender (adjective) - Global term used to describe people whose gender identity does not coincide with the sex and gender assigned to them at birth and/or people whose gender is nonconforming or whose gender expression does not fit the typical definition of feminine or masculine.

Transgender female (adjective) (may be described as MtF, male to female) - A person with a feminine gender identity that does not correspond to the sex and gender assigned at birth (male).

Transgender male (adjective) (may be described as FtM, female to male) - A person with a masculine gender identity that does not correspond to the sex and gender assigned at birth (female).

About the Author

Ana Macedo, 51 years old, 5 children, physician, graduated in 1997 from the University of Lisbon School of Medicine. PhD in Pharmacology from the Autonomous University of Barcelona. Academic title of aggregation from the University of the Algarve.

Currently she is an Invited Associate Professor with Aggregation at the Faculty of Medicine and Biomedical Sciences at the University of Algarve. Director of the PhD Program in Clinical Research and Translational Medicine at the University of Algarve. Chair of the Ethics Committee of the Algarve Biomedical Center.

Author of the books, ' No Patient Left Behind: A Comprehensive Guide to Inclusive Clinical Research', 'Como Nascem Novos Medicamentos', 'Estatística Precisa-se'. 'A Saúde não ter Preço mas tem Custos'.

www.anamacedo.pt

www.ingramcontent.com/pod-product-compliance
Lightning Source LLC
Chambersburg PA
CBHW050210230526
45470CB00001B/322